Latest Breakthroughs in the Treatment of Atopic Dermatitis

Edited by Charbel Skayem and Tu Anh Duong

Published in London, United Kingdom

Latest Breakthroughs in the Treatment of Atopic Dermatitis
http://dx.doi.org/10.5772/intechopen.104344
Edited by Charbel Skayem and Tu Anh Duong

Contributors
Charbel Skayem, Tu Anh Duong, Leisheng Zhang, Xiaonan Yang, Zhihai Han, Zhongchao Han, Tiankang Guo, Xiaowei Gao, Hui Cai, Ewa J. Kleczyk, Julie Mallory Crawford, Laura Dalfonso, Rosanna Marsella

First published in London, United Kingdom, 2024 by IntechOpen
IntechOpen is the global imprint of INTECHOPEN LIMITED, registered in England and Wales, registration number: 11086078, 5 Princes Gate Court, London, SW7 2QJ, United Kingdom

British Library Cataloguing-in-Publication Data
A catalogue record for this book is available from the British Library

Additional hard and PDF copies can be obtained from orders@intechopen.com

Latest Breakthroughs in the Treatment of Atopic Dermatitis
Edited by Charbel Skayem and Tu Anh Duong
p. cm.
Print ISBN 978-1-83769-514-0
Online ISBN 978-1-83769-513-3
eBook (PDF) ISBN 978-1-83769-515-7

For EU product safety concerns:
IN TECH d.o.o., Prolaz Marije Krucifikse Kozulić 3, 51000 Rijeka, Croatia,
info@intechopen.com or visit our website at intechopen.com.

Meet the editor

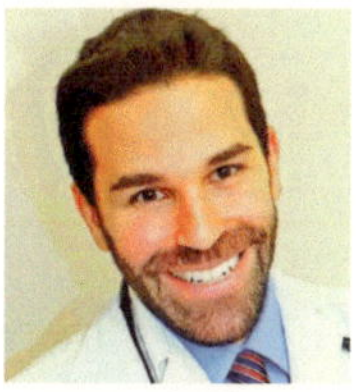

Dr. Charbel Skayem is a dermatologist, venereologist, and dermatologic surgeon practicing in Assistance Publique des Hôpitaux de Paris (AP-HP), the largest university hospital system in Europe and one of the largest in the world, and in Gustave Roussy, the first cancer-research hospital in Europe and among the top three specialized university hospitals in the world. Lebanese in origin, he moved to Paris to pursue his residency in dermatology and venereology, followed by several fellowships, graduating from the Sorbonne University, the University of Paris, and Paris-Saclay University. His initial experiences in different world-renowned pioneer referral departments have given him wide expertise in multiple branches of his specialty, including oncodermatology, advanced dermatologic surgery, inflammatory and infectious dermatology, teledermatology, sexually transmitted diseases, and cosmetic and laser dermatology. Dr Skayem is a member of different dermatological societies and academies. He was a laureate of several scholarships and awards. He was a distinguished speaker at many global congresses. Despite his youth, he has served as a reviewer and editor, writing several book chapters and articles in leading peer-reviewed medical journals.

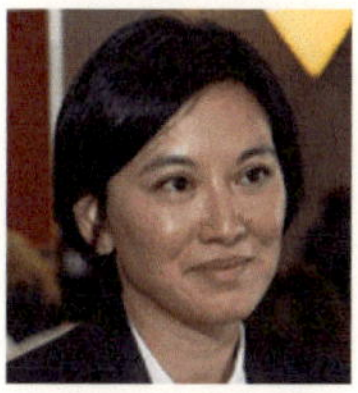

Dr. Tu Anh Duong is a dermatologist in Assistance Publique des Hôpitaux de Paris (AP-HP), the largest hospital system in Europe, Paris-Saclay University, and a numeric design engineer in medicine. Affiliated to leading referral departments in dermatology (in toxic epidermal necrolysis, bullous dermatological diseases, severe cutaneous adverse reactions, dermatological emergencies, and neurofibromatosis), Dr. Duong has wide expertise in severe skin disorders. She is an innovator in the field of teledermatology and is the president of teledermatology in the French Society of Dermatology, the coordinator of TELDERM AP-HP, and Chair of Avenir Santé Numérique. Her innovations and interests lie in dermatological emergencies and engineering dermatological numeric transformations and conversions. Dr. Duong is the author of hundreds of articles in leading peer-reviewed medical journals.

Contents

Preface **IX**

Chapter 1 **1**
Introductory Chapter: Deciphering Complexities of Atopic Dermatitis Shifts Paradigms in Treatment
by Charbel Skayem and Tu Anh Duong

Chapter 2 **5**
Natural Killer Cells in Atopic Dermatitis Opening Doors to New Treatments
by Leisheng Zhang, Xiaonan Yang, Zhihai Han, Zhongchao Han, Tiankang Guo, Xiaowei Gao and Hui Cai

Chapter 3 **17**
Leveraging Disease-Based Community Data to Provide Insights into Current Atopic Dermatitis Treatments
by Ewa J. Kleczyk, Julie Mallory Crawford and Laura Dalfonso

Chapter 4 **33**
An Era of Therapeutic Evolution and Revolution: Insights into Studies on Dupilumab, Tralokinumab, Lebrikizumab, Nemolizumab, Eblasakimab, and OX40/OX40L Agents (Rocatinlimab and Amlitelimab) in Moderate-to-Severe Atopic Dermatitis
by Charbel Skayem and Tu Anh Duong

Chapter 5 **43**
New Treatments and Validations for Atopic Dermatitis in Humans after Comparative Approach with Canine Models
by Rosanna Marsella

Preface

Despite being a common chronic inflammatory skin disease, atopic dermatitis (AD) has been poorly understood throughout history. However, the last decade has witnessed an unprecedented pace of change; we were able to decrypt the cellular and molecular intricacies of this disease and develop new drugs that target specific interleukins implicated in its pathophysiology. This gives the potential for a precision medicine approach that enables more effective long-term control of this complex disease. This book highlights the latest breakthroughs in the understanding of AD and the novel agents currently being investigated for treatment.

Charbel Skayem
Faculty of Medicine,
Sorbonne University,
Paris, France

Paris Saclay University Hôpitaux de Paris (AP-HP),
Paris, France

Tu Anh Duong
Telemedicine Department,
Assistance Publique Hôpitaux de Paris (AP-HP),
Paris Saclay University,
Paris, France

Chapter 1

Introductory Chapter: Deciphering Complexities of Atopic Dermatitis Shifts Paradigms in Treatment

Charbel Skayem and Tu Anh Duong

1. Introduction

Atopic dermatitis (AD) in adults can either be a relapsing form of childhood AD or a new adult-onset, the latter being less common. However, the diagnosis of adult-onset AD should be made with caution, as numerous skin conditions may present as eczematous dermatitis in adulthood. Patients who are not eligible or do not respond to intensive topical therapy or phototherapy require systemic therapies [1]. Recent advancements in understanding AD pathogenesis resulted in a real translational revolution and led to the exponential expansion of the therapeutic pipeline. Focusing on biomarkers in emerging treatment studies clarifies the role of each cytokine and immune pathway. Moreover, it allows us to address the unique immune fingerprints of each AD subset. In the future, personalized medicine will be the ultimate goal of this targeted translational research [2]. With the changes in the concepts of both the pathogenesis and treatment approach to AD and the breadth of management options available, choosing the appropriate systemic therapy is becoming challenging.

2. Approach to management of severe atopic dermatitis

There are several factors to consider before starting a systemic treatment in adults with severe AD. To begin with, identifying the causes of recalcitrant disease seems mandatory.

These include lack of adherence to treatment, coexisting allergic contact dermatitis, or photosensitive dermatitis, secondary infection, and vitamin D deficiency.

The lack of practicality of topical treatment leads to decreased adherence over time and persistent disease. Moreover, concerns about adverse effects, like corticosteroid phobia, may lead to inadequate application [1, 3].

Decolonization of staphylococcal aureus infections should be considered in case of recurrent episodes. Chlorhexidine showers, nasal mupirocin, and frequent bathing with or without bleach can help reduce carriage. Family members or cohabitating individuals are often carriers; therefore, treatment of the whole housing unit can stop recurrent infections [4].

Concurrent allergic contact dermatitis has to be considered in all patients with severe AD. Patients have to be patch-tested before being placed on

IntechOpen

immunosuppressants to avoid false-negative results. Allergens in many topical over-the-counter or prescribed products as well as other common allergens, can all complicate AD [5–9].

The decision to start systemic therapies is based upon consideration of patient's adherence to topical therapies, disease severity, frequency of flares, and impact on the patient's quality of life.

In clinical practice, in addition to visually evaluating the severity and extent of AD, clinicians may assess the impact of the diseases on patients' quality of life by asking open-ended questions on the intensity of symptoms, frequency of flares, and impact of disease on daily activities, psychosocial life, and sleep. The burden of treatment, including time spent on treatment, cost of medications, and frequency of physician visits, should be assessed as well.

3. Indications of systemic therapy in AD

Several disease severity scales for AD have been validated. However, they are not commonly used in clinical practice and may not accurately identify those in need of systemic therapies. These include: SCORAD (Scoring Atopic Dermatitis), EASI (Eczema Area and Severity Index), POEM (Patient-Oriented Eczema Measure), and DLQI (Dermatology Life Quality Index).

In fact, systemic therapy is required in patients who are not candidates or do not respond to intensive topical therapy or phototherapy.

The main goals of therapy are the improvement of signs and symptoms as well as the overall quality of life.

Over the past decade, our understanding of the pathophysiology and clinical burden of AD has rapidly evolved, with a dramatic increase in new systemic therapies.

While current data is highly promising, supplemental clinical trials are still needed to further elucidate the long-term safety, efficacy, and durability of these treatments. Moreover, comparison studies are also needed to better orient physicians in their choice of systemic therapy [1].

Finally, the combination of clinical efficacy in clinical trials with biomarkers and mechanistic studies has helped select the most promising molecules and will shape the direction of future research. This translational revolution could lead to predicting patients' responses to targeted therapy, thus guiding the choice of the most suitable treatment.

Author details

Charbel Skayem[1,2]* and Tu Anh Duong[3,4,5]

1 Faculty of Medicine, Sorbonne University, Paris, France

2 Paris Saclay University, Hôpitaux de Paris (AP-HP), Paris, France

3 Telemedicine Department, Paris Saclay University, Assistance Publique Hôpitaux de Paris (AP-HP), Paris, France

4 Chaire Avenir Santé numérique, Paris, France

5 Research Group Dynamyc, Paris, France

*Address all correspondence to: charbelskayem@hotmail.com

References

[1] Berger T. Evaluation and management of severe refractory atopic dermatitis (eczema) in adults. Uptodate. 16 Jun 2023

[2] Facheris P, Jeffery J, Del Duca E, Guttman-Yassky E. The translational revolution in atopic dermatitis: The paradigm shift from pathogenesis to treatment. Cellular & Molecular Immunology. May 2023;**20**(5):448-474. DOI: 10.1038/s41423-023-00992-4. Epub 2023 Mar 16. PMID: 36928371; PMCID: PMC10203371

[3] Li AW, Yin ES, Antaya RJ. Topical corticosteroid phobia in atopic dermatitis: A systematic review. JAMA Dermatology. 2017;**153**:1036

[4] Chopra R, Vakharia PP, Sacotte R, Silverberg JI. Efficacy of bleach baths in reducing severity of atopic dermatitis: A systematic review and meta-analysis. Annals of Allergy, Asthma & Immunology. 2017;**119**:435

[5] Drucker AM, Morra DE, Prieto-Merino D, et al. Systemic immunomodulatory treatments for atopic dermatitis: Update of a living systematic review and network meta-analysis. JAMA Dermatology. 2022;**158**(5):523-532. DOI: 10.1001/jamadermatol.2022.0455

[6] Kim JP, Chao LX, Simpson EL, Silverberg JI. Persistence of atopic dermatitis (AD): A systematic review and meta-analysis. Journal of the American Academy of Dermatology. Oct 2016;**75**(4):681-687.e11. DOI: 10.1016/j.jaad.2016.05.028. Epub 2016 Aug 17. PMID: 27544489; PMCID: PMC5216177

[7] Simpson EL, Bruin-Weller M, Flohr C, Ardern-Jones MR, Barbarot S, Deleuran M, et al. When does atopic dermatitis warrant systemic therapy? Recommendations from an expert panel of the International Eczema Council. Journal of the American Academy of Dermatology. Oct 2017;**77**(4):623-633. DOI: 10.1016/j.jaad.2017.06.042. Epub 2017 Aug 10. PMID: 28803668

[8] Schneider S, Li L, Zink A. The new era of biologics in atopic dermatitis: A review. Dermatology Practical & Conceptual. 1 Oct 2021;**11**(4):e2021144. DOI: 10.5826/dpc.1104a144. PMCID: PMC8648434

[9] Yamamura K, Nakahara T. The Dawn of a new era in atopic dermatitis treatment. Journal of Clinical Medicine. Oct 2022;**11**(20):6145. DOI: 10.3390/jcm11206145. PMID: 36294465; PMCID: PMC9605067

Chapter 2

Natural Killer Cells in Atopic Dermatitis Opening Doors to New Treatments

Leisheng Zhang, Xiaonan Yang, Zhihai Han, Zhongchao Han, Tiankang Guo, Xiaowei Gao and Hui Cai

Abstract

Longitudinal studies have indicated the multifaceted regimens for atopic dermatitis (AD) administration, including ultraviolet phototherapy, oral JAK inhibitors, and the concomitant adjunctive therapies according to the American Academy of Dermatology published Guidelines of Care for the Management of Atopic Dermatitis. As a disease with typical characteristics of relapsing pruritus and chronic inflammation, AD has caused heavy burden on children and adults, as well as healthcare providers and family members. As a multi-factorial disease, AD has been considered primarily derived by Th2 dysfunction, with clinical and molecular heterogeneity. The current therapeutic regimens are various and largely due to the diversity in the wide spectrum of the clinical phenotypes based on epidermal barrier disruption, genetic predisposition, and dysregulation of patients' immune system. Meanwhile there's an urgent need for developing safer and long-term agents to efficiently control moderate to severe AD. In this book chapter, we mainly summarized the fundamental concept, clinical manifestation, pathophysiology and molecular mechanisms of AD, and in particular, the biofunction and modulation of natural killer (NK) cells for AD. Collectively, the contents in this chapter will help further understand the landscape of this disease and the rationale behind new emerging therapies.

Keywords: natural killer cells, atopic dermatitis, pathogenesis, pathophysiology, clinical trials

1. Introduction

As an extremely heterogeneous disease with varying phenotypes, AD has caused overwhelming pain to the patients and the guardians physically and mentally as well as significant incidence and healthcare costs [1–4]. For decades, AD has been proved with the occurrence in childhood and the increased incidence rate with age, which also increases the risk of allergic rhinitis, food allergy, and asthma later in life as well [5]. For example, patients with AD should continuously suffer xerosis (dry skin) and the intensely pruritic lesions spread all over the body [6]. As reviewed by Napolitano and the colleagues, AD in adults and adolescents can be divided into several subtypes, including the head and neck eczema, the flexural eczema, the hand eczema, erythrodermia (0.7%), diffuse eczema (6.5%), portrait-like dermatitis (20.1%), prurigo nodularis-like dermatitis (2.1%), and eczema nummulare-like dermatitis (5.8%) [7]. On the one hand, the criteria for clinical diagnosis of AD mainly contain the albeit with age-related differences and the typically distributed eczematous lesions in AD patients [7]. On the other hand, the most effective options of AD administration are aiming to decrease inflammation and restore the skin barrier [5].

State-of-the-art renewal has indicated the involvement of T lymphocytes, natural killer (NK) cells and dendritic cells (DCs) as well as invariant natural killer T (iNKT) cells for the pathogenesis of the complex inflammatory cutaneous disorder via mediating the inflammatory reaction and the epidermal barrier dysfunction as well [8–13]. For example, the genetic predisposition of atopics in AD patients is caused by the expansion of Th2 cells and mast cells as well as the release of eosinophilia-associated cytokines (e.g., IL-3, IL-4, IL-5, and IL-13) and IgE [14, 15]. Meanwhile, Ilhan et al. verified that AD patients revealed decline in the proportion of Valpha24$^+$CD161$^+$ NKT cell subtypes compared with the corresponding healthy individuals, whereas no differ was observed in the CD3$^+$CD16$^+$CD56$^+$ NKT cell counterpart [16]. As reviewed by von Bubnoff and the colleagues, NK cells have been considered as the known immune deviation for AD via contributing the production of Th2 cytokines (e.g., IFN-gamma), whereas Luci *et al* reported the qualitative and quantitative alterations of peripheral NK cells in AD patients [17, 18].

For the purpose, in this book chapter, we mainly focus on the rudimentary knowledge of AD from the aspects of clinical diagnosis, pathophysiology, molecular mechanisms, and systemic therapy of AD, which will benefit the further understanding of the pathogenesis of AD and the concomitant dysfunction of NK cells for the common chronic inflammatory skin disease and facilitating the personalized and targeted therapy in future.

2. Atopic dermatitis

Atopic dermatitis (AD), also known as atopic eczema, has been recognized as a global health issue with pruritus as the primary lesion [19, 20]. For decades, AD has caused extensive burden on children and adults, whereas the extent and appearance of lesions vary with race and age [21]. Currently, AD patients are considered with a family or personal history of atopic disease, which occupy a percentage of approximately 75–80% of the total AD cases [22]. Meanwhile, AD is commonly complicated by allergic rhinitis, asthma, and food allergies as well, which further aggravates the complexity and the difficulty of treatment upon AD [3].

Worse still, the dermatologic manifestations of AD are also diverse in clinical presentations, which are detrimental to disease diagnosis in clinical practice. Generally, the clinical manifestations of AD contain atopy and pruritus, which is triggered by a variety of irritants including Soaps, detergents, disinfectants, occupational chemicals, fumes, Juices from fresh fruits, meats, vegetables, house dust mites, pets (e.g., cats, dogs, birds), pollens (seasonal), molds, human dander, Staph Aureus, viral infections, mycologic pityrosporum, candida, dermatophytes, temperature/climate, foods (e.g., irritant, vasodilators, allergen), psyche, and hormones [14]. In brief, as summarized by Beltrani et al., AD and the concomitant clinical presentations and course were considered as a syndrome constituted by an identifiable group of symptoms and signs representing the multidimensional dermatological manifestation of atopic diathesis [14]. For decades, we and other investigators in the field are dedicating to verify the pathophysiology and the underlying pathogenesis of AD to incorporate novel treatments in both preclinical and clinical practice. Meanwhile, a range of academic organizations have also published a number of guidelines for AD diagnosis and treatment, such as "Guidelines of Care for the Management of Atopic Dermatitis" published by the American Academy of Dermatology and the document entitled "Japanese guidelines for atopic dermatitis 2017" released by the Japanese Society of Allergology [23, 24].

2.1 Pathophysiology of atopic dermatitis

Despite the incompletely understood of the etiology due to the complicated and multifactorial pathogenesis of AD, the pathophysiology of AD is continuously explored and uncovered, and in particular, the interaction among immune dysfunction, genetic predisposition, and the environmental provocation factors for AD development [4, 25]. In details, the pathophysiology of AD is multifactorial and complex, including the alterations in cell mediated immune responses, dehydration, the elements of barrier dysfunction, environmental factors, pH alterations, increase in the trans-epidermal water loss, and the IgE mediated hypersensitivity [26, 27]. For example, the environmental pollutants and the concomitant diverse environmental factors appear to accelerate the occurrence of AD via triggering responses from both the adaptive and innate immune pathways, such as harsh detergents, airborne formaldehyde, preservatives, and fragrances. To date, a variety of molecular biomarkers have been identified to play a role in different ways, such as measuring treatment response, predicting clinical prognosis, and gauging disease severity [1]. Currently, phototherapy is the major and effective therapeutic modality for various skin diseases, including AD, eczema, photodermatitis, vitiligo, parapsoriasis, and psoriasis, yet the outcomes of AD patients are not satisfactory and persistent [28]. Therefore, based on the indicated biomarkers, novel therapeutic options are hopefully developed for AD patients, and in particular, the targeted and individualized immunomodulators for AD administration.

At the meantime, current advances in the aforementioned pathophysiology of AD are facilitating the stratification of different AD phenotypes, which thus would potentially convert to the development of targeted-specific, personalized regimens of AD in future [29, 30]. State-of-the-art literatures have indicated the feasibility of effective strategies for the improvement of AD, including detailed countermeasures and investigation of the potential causes and the exacerbating factors, correction of skin dysfunctions in AD patients, and the concomitant pharmacotherapy [19, 24].

2.2 Molecular mechanisms of atopic dermatitis

To date, a variety of elements have been considered to play a role during the development of AD [31]. For example, the imbalance of Th1 and Th2 is adequate to increase alterations in cell mediated immune responses and thus facilitate IgE-mediated hypersensitivity [26]. For example, T lymphocytes have been supposed to be the principal effector cells of various eczematous conditions, yet a number of infiltration patterns of T-cell subsets with significant differences are also noted in AD, and in particular, the ratio of $CD4^+$ T helper cells and the $CD8^+$ T suppressor cells is higher in the papillary dermal infiltrate but lower in the epidermal infiltration [14]. Meanwhile, Jensen et al. found that patients with moderate to severe atopic dermatitis revealed reduced NK cell activity and enhanced effect of IFN-γ [32]. Therewith, verification of the numerous and complex changes of the innate and adaptive immunity at both the phenotypic level and the genetic level will collectively provide the basis for dissecting the various endotypes and phenotypes of AD and developing novel systemic intervention [33].

Overall, AD has been considered with association with the NK cell-mediated immune dysregulation attributes to the direct interaction of NK cells with the polymorphic HLA class I (HLA-I) ligand variants via the killer cell Ig-like receptors (KIRs, such as KIR2DL5, KIR2DS5, and KIR2DS1), [34–37]. Taken together, systematic and detailed verification of the molecular mechanisms of AD via underpinning the epidermal barrier dysfunction will resultant in a better comprehension of the pathophysiological mechanisms of AD and the complications [3].

3. Natural killer (NK) cells

Natural killer (NK) cells are heterogeneous lymphocytes generated from hematopoietic stem cells (HSCs), which is firstly identified by Kiessling et al. in the 1970s [38, 39]. NK cells belong to the third type of lymphocytes, which are distinguish from the T lymphocytes and B lymphocytes [18, 40–42]. For example, NK cells play a critical role in both innate immune and adaptive immune dispense with the requirement of prior sensitization as well as the recognition of peptide antigens. Compared with the chimeric antigen receptor-transduced T (CAR-T) cells, NK cells display excellent cytotoxic effect via both the receptor-dependent and receptor-independent signaling cascades by orchestrating the molecular mechanisms including antibody-dependent cell-mediated cytotoxicity (ADCC), paracrine effects (e.g., TNF-α, IFN-γ, GM-CSF), direct cytolytic effect, and the manipulation of relative immune contextures [39, 43–46]. Meanwhile, the potent adverse reaction and immune-related adverse events (irAEs) of CAR-T cells can be efficiently avoided in NK cell-based immunotherapy, such as acute graft-versus-host disease (aGvHD), cytokine release syndrome (CRS), and immune cell- associated neurotoxicity syndrome (iCANS) [39, 47–49].

Generally, NK cells can be enriched from a variety of sources, such as peripheral blood, umbilical cord blood, placental blood, NK cell lines (e.g., NK-92MI, YT), and stem cells including hematopoietic stem cells (HSCs), induced pluripotent stem cells (iPSCs) and embryonic stem cells (ESCs) [39, 50–52]. For example, in peripheral blood, NK cells occupy a percentage of 5–20% of leukocytes, including the $CD56^{dim}CD16^{high}$ subpopulation and the $CD56^{bright}CD16^{low/neg}$ counterpart [39, 53]. NK cells are acknowledged for the unique ability to recognize and kill tumor cells via the secretion of cytokines and direct interaction. NK cells exert cytotoxicity against pathogenic microorganism, tumor cells, infected cells and aging cells [54]. Meanwhile, NK cells are adequate to modulate the biofunction of relative immune cells via direct cell-cell contact-dependent mode and secretion of chemokines, cytokines, granuloenzyme and perforin [40, 55].

Nowadays, circulating NK cells in the peripheral blood have been considered with altered function and reduced frequency in individuals with moderate-to-severe AD, which suggests the potential feasibility of the immunotherapy strategy for AD administration [18, 56, 57]. Interestingly, the overactivation of NK cells has been found in patients with pemphigus vulgaris and alopecia areata as well as AD [18]. For example, NK cells are adequate to collaborate with type 2 immune cells for the modulation of the pathogenesis of AD [58]. Because interferon-γ (IFN-γ) generated by NK cells and the relative immune cell types is considered as a prominent modulator for negative regulation of the aforementioned type 2 immunity. Notably, Alkon and the colleagues took advantage of the single-cell RNA-SEQ analysis and identified the innate lymphoid cell (ILC) lineage infidelity in AD. In details, they found that the majority of cutaneous ILCs between AD and normal human skin (NHS) belonged to the $CRTH2^+$ subpopulation and these cells resided in the upper skin layers [59]. Instead, Min verified that the $CD1d^{hi}PD\text{-}L1^{hi}CD27^+$ regulatory NK cell subset could efficiently suppress AD via significantly inhibiting the numbers of ILC2s and Th2 cells, which collectively suggested the biofunction and association of TGF-β-producing NK cells with the severity of AD [60].

According to the ClinicalTrials.gov (https://www.clinicaltrials.gov/) website, there are a total number of 5 trials upon NK cells and AD, including 3 observational trials (NCT04354207, NCT01429311, NCT03581747) and 2 interventional trials (NCT00824889, NCT02564055), which is distributed in Lithuania, United States, France, Switzerland (**Figure 1**, **Table 1**). As mentioned above, the detailed information of NK cells in the pathogenesis and therapy of AD is still far from satisfactory.

4. Discussion and conclusions

AD has caused unbearable pain to numerous patients and their companions, and there's an urgent demand for the development of effective, well tolerated, and personalized treatment regimens in the near future. Natural killer (NK) cells are lymphocytes involved in both innate immune response and adaptive immune response, which are also considered with pathogenicity during AD and thus provide novel candidates

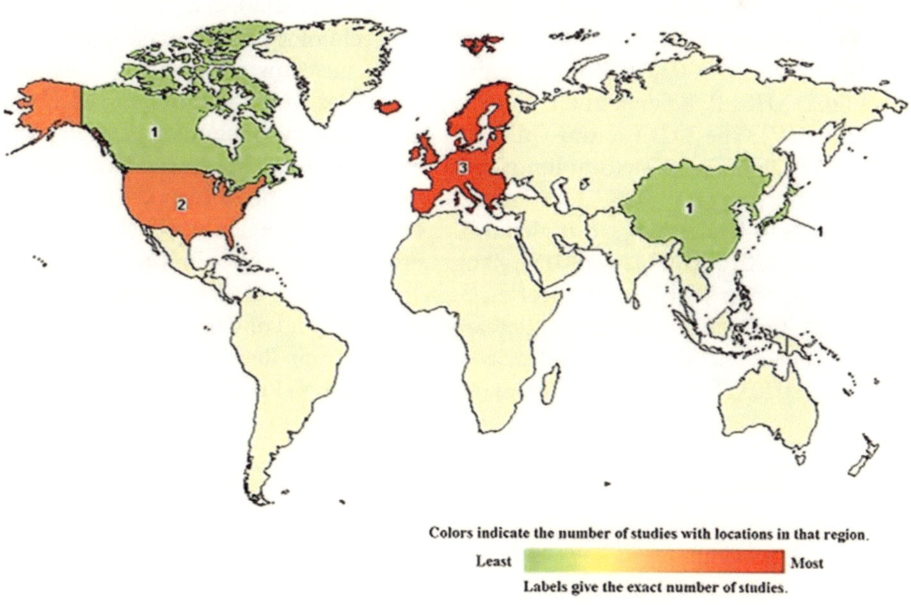

Figure 1.
The map of clinical trials upon AD and NK cells.

NCT Number	Study Type	Enrollment	Locations
NCT04354207	Observational	500	Lithuania
NCT01429311	Observational	84	United States
NCT00824889	Interventional	28	France
NCT03581747	Observational	1000	Switzerland
NCT02564055	Interventional	247	United States

Table 1.
Clinical trials of NK cells for AD.

for establishing the aforementioned well tolerated and personalized therapeutic schedules of atopic dermatitis in future.

Acknowledgements

The coauthors thank the members in NHC Key Laboratory of Diagnosis and Therapy of Gastrointestinal Tumor & Key Laboratory of Molecular Diagnostics and Precision Medicine for Surgical Oncology in Gansu Province, Gansu Provincial Hospital, Hefei Institute of Physical Science in Chinese Academy of Sciences, The First Affiliated Hospital of Shandong First Medical University, and Health-Biotech (Tianjin) Stem Cell Research Institute Co., Ltd., and Jiangxi Health-Biotech Stem Cell Technology Co., Ltd. for their technical support. This work was supported by grants from the National Natural Science Foundation of China (No. 82260031), the project Youth Fund supported by Shandong Provincial Natural Science Foundation (ZR2020QC097), Natural Science Foundation of Jiangxi Province (20224BAB206077, 20212BAB216073), Key Project funded by Department of Science and Technology of Shangrao City (2020AB002, 2022AB003, 2022A001), Fujian Provincial Ministerial Finance Special Project (2021XH018), Science and technology projects of Guizhou Province (QKH-J-ZK[2021]-107), The 2021 Central-Guided Local Science and Technology Development Fund (ZYYDDFFZZJ-1), Medical Innovation Project of Fujian Provincial Health and Health Commission (2019-CX-21), Natural Science Foundation of Jiangxi Province (20212BAB216073), Key project funded by Department of Science and Technology of Shangrao City (2020 K003, 2021F013), Jiangxi Provincial Key New Product Incubation Program Funded by Technical Innovation Guidance Program of Shangrao City (2020G002), the Non-profit Central Research Institute Fund of Chinese Academy of Medical Sciences (2019PT320005), Horizontal Project upon Retrospective Analyses of COVID-19 (2020XH001), Double Thousand Plan of Jiangxi Province (2022 to LSZ).

Conflict of interest

The authors declare no conflict of interest.

Notes/thanks/other declarations

Not applicable.

Appendices and nomenclature

ADCC	antibody-dependent cell-mediated cytotoxicity
hPSCs	human pluripotent stem cells
NK	natural killer
hESCs	human embryonic stem cells
hiPSCs	human inducible pluripotent stem cells
UCB	umbilical cord blood
PB	peripheral blood
PBMCs	peripheral blood-derived mononuclear cells
PB-NK	peripheral blood-derived NK
IFN-γ	interferon-γ
AD	atopic dermatitis
aGvHD	acute graft-versus-host disease
irAEs	immune-related adverse events
HSCs	hematopoietic stem cells
CRS	cytokine release syndrome
aGvHD	acute graft-versus-host disease
iCANS	immune cell-associated neurotoxicity syndrome
CAR-T	chimeric antigen receptor-transduced T
NK	natural killer
ADCC	antibody-dependent cell-mediated cytotoxicity
DCs	dendritic cells
iNKT	invariant natural killer T

Author details

Leisheng Zhang[1,2,3,4,5*†], Xiaonan Yang[6†], Zhihai Han[4], Zhongchao Han[3,4,7], Tiankang Guo[1*], Xiaowei Gao[8*] and Hui Cai[1*]

1 Key Laboratory of Molecular Diagnostics and Precision Medicine for Surgical Oncology in Gansu Province and NHC Key Laboratory of Diagnosis and Therapy of Gastrointestinal Tumor, Gansu Provincial Hospital, China

2 Key Laboratory of Radiation Technology and Biophysics, Hefei Institutes of Physical Science, Chinese Academy of Sciences, China

3 Institute of Health-Biotech, Health-Biotech (Tianjin) Stem Cell Research Institute Co., Ltd., China

4 Jiangxi Research Center of Stem Cell Engineering, Jiangxi Health-Biotech Stem Cell Technology Co., Ltd., China

5 Center for Cellular Therapies, The First Affiliated Hospital of Shandong First Medical University, China

6 Department of Plastic and Reconstructive Surgery and Department of Hemangioma and Vescular Malformation, Plastic Surgery Hospital Affiliated to Chinese Academy of Medical Sciences and Peking Union Medical College, China

7 State Key Laboratory of Experimental Hematology, National Clinical Research Center for Blood Diseases, Haihe Laboratory of Cell Ecosystem, Institute of Hematology and Blood Diseases Hospital, Chinese Academy of Medical Sciences & Peking Union Medical College, Tianjin, China

8 Department of Otorhinolaryngology, Second Hospital of Tianjin Medical University, Tianjin, China

*Address all correspondence to: leisheng_zhang@163.com; tiankangguo2020@163.com; beny51@126.com and caialonteam@163.com

† Co-first author.

References

[1] Hassan S, Hamideh N, Poulos C, Cheema S, Rangwani S, Lio PA. Atopic dermatitis biomarkers and the movement toward personalized treatment. Dermatitis. 2021;**32**(1S):S8-S14

[2] Jurakic Toncic R, Marinovic B. The role of impaired epidermal barrier function in atopic dermatitis. Acta Dermatovenerologica Croatica. 2016;**24**(2):95-109

[3] Kubo A, Nagao K, Amagai M. Epidermal barrier dysfunction and cutaneous sensitization in atopic diseases. The Journal of Clinical Investigation. 2012;**122**(2):440-447

[4] Yue H, Umehara Y, Trujillo-Paez JV, Peng G, Nguyen HLT, Chieosilapatham P, et al. Exogenous factors in the pathogenesis of atopic dermatitis: Irritants and cutaneous infections. Clinical and Experimental Allergy. 2021;**51**(3):382-392

[5] Kraft MT, Prince BT. Atopic dermatitis is a barrier issue, not an allergy issue. Immunology and Allergy Clinics of North America. 2019;**39**(4):507-519

[6] Johnson KM, Will BM, Johnson DW. Diagnosis and management of atopic dermatitis. JAAPA. 2021;**34**(7):32-36

[7] Napolitano M, Fabbrocini G, Martora F, Genco L, Noto M, Patruno C. Children atopic dermatitis: Diagnosis, mimics, overlaps, and therapeutic implication. Dermatologic Therapy. 2022;**35**(12):e15901

[8] Guttman-Yassky E, Waldman A, Ahluwalia J, Ong PY, Eichenfield LF. Atopic dermatitis: Pathogenesis. Seminars in Cutaneous Medicine and Surgery. 2017;**36**(3):100-103

[9] Santos LS, Sgnotto FDR, Sousa TR, Orfali RL, Aoki V, Duarte A, et al. IgG from atopic dermatitis patients induces non-atopic infant thymic invariant natural killer T (iNKT) cells to produce IL-4, IL-17, and IL-10. International Journal of Dermatology. 2020;**59**(3):359-364

[10] Kabashima K, Weidinger S. NK cells as a possible new player in atopic dermatitis. The Journal of Allergy and Clinical Immunology. 2020;**146**(2):276-277

[11] Gyimesi E, Nagy G, Remenyik E, Sipka S, Zeher M, Biro T, et al. Altered peripheral invariant natural killer T cells in atopic dermatitis. Journal of Clinical Immunology. 2011;**31**(5):864-872

[12] Worm M, Glatzel V, Baumgart S, Mei HE, Sorensen T, Grutzkau A, et al. Immune cell profiling reveals natural killer and T cell subpopulations to be associated with atopic dermatitis severity. Clinical and Experimental Allergy. 2023;**53**(1):105-108

[13] Buentke E, Heffler LC, Wilson JL, Wallin RP, Lofman C, Chambers BJ, et al. Natural killer and dendritic cell contact in lesional atopic dermatitis skin--Malassezia-influenced cell interaction. The Journal of Investigative Dermatology. 2002;**119**(4):850-857

[14] Beltrani VS, Boguneiwicz M. Atopic dermatitis. Dermatology Online Journal. 2003;**9**(2):1

[15] Mobus L, Rodriguez E, Harder I, Boraczynski N, Szymczak S, Hubenthal M, et al. Blood transcriptome

profiling identifies 2 candidate endotypes of atopic dermatitis. The Journal of Allergy and Clinical Immunology. 2022;**150**(2):385-395

[16] Ilhan F, Kandi B, Akbulut H, Turgut D, Cicek D. Atopic dermatitis and Valpha24+ natural killer T cells. Skinmed. 2007;**6**(5):218-220

[17] Luci C, Gaudy-Marqueste C, Rouzaire P, Audonnet S, Cognet C, Hennino A, et al. Peripheral natural killer cells exhibit qualitative and quantitative changes in patients with psoriasis and atopic dermatitis. The British Journal of Dermatology. 2012;**166**(4):789-796

[18] von Bubnoff D, Andres E, Hentges F, Bieber T, Michel T, Zimmer J. Natural killer cells in atopic and autoimmune diseases of the skin. The Journal of Allergy and Clinical Immunology. 2010;**125**(1):60-68

[19] Katoh N, Ohya Y, Ikeda M, Ebihara T, Katayama I, Saeki H, et al. Japanese guidelines for atopic dermatitis 2020. Allergology International. 2020;**69**(3):356-369

[20] Waldman AR, Ahluwalia J, Udkoff J, Borok JF, Eichenfield LF. Atopic Dermatitis. Pediatrics in Review. 2018;**39**(4):180-193

[21] Stander S. Atopic Dermatitis. The New England Journal of Medicine. 2021;**384**(12):1136-1143

[22] Borirakchanyavat K, Kurban AK. Atopic dermatitis. Clinics in Dermatology. 2000;**18**(6):649-655

[23] Sidbury R, Kodama S. Atopic dermatitis guidelines: Diagnosis, systemic therapy, and adjunctive care. Clinics in Dermatology. 2018;**36**(5):648-652

[24] Katayama I, Aihara M, Ohya Y, Saeki H, Shimojo N, Shoji S, et al. Japanese society of A: Japanese guidelines for atopic dermatitis 2017. Allergology International. 2017;**66**(2):230-247

[25] Mobus L, Rodriguez E, Harder I, Stolzl D, Boraczynski N, Gerdes S, et al. Atopic dermatitis displays stable and dynamic skin transcriptome signatures. The Journal of Allergy and Clinical Immunology. 2021;**147**(1):213-223

[26] David Boothe W, Tarbox JA, Tarbox MB. Atopic dermatitis: Pathophysiology. Advances in Experimental Medicine and Biology. 2017;**1027**:21-37

[27] Damour A, Garcia M, Seneschal J, Leveque N, Bodet C. Eczema herpeticum: Clinical and pathophysiological aspects. Clinical Reviews in Allergy and Immunology. 2020;**59**(1):1-18

[28] Rathod DG, Muneer H, Masood S. Phototherapy. Treasure Island (FL): StatPearls; 2022

[29] Cabanillas B, Brehler AC, Novak N. Atopic dermatitis phenotypes and the need for personalized medicine. Current Opinion in Allergy and Clinical Immunology. 2017;**17**(4):309-315

[30] Traidl S, Roesner L, Zeitvogel J, Werfel T. Eczema herpeticum in atopic dermatitis. Allergy. 2021;**76**(10):3017-3027

[31] Fabrazzo M, Cipolla S, Signoriello S, Camerlengo A, Calabrese G, Giordano GM, et al. A systematic review on shared biological mechanisms of depression and anxiety in comorbidity with psoriasis, atopic dermatitis, and hidradenitis suppurativa. European Psychiatry. 2021;**64**(1):e71

[32] Jensen JR, Sand TT, Jorgensen AS, Thestrup-Pedersen K. Modulation of natural killer cell activity in patients with atopic dermatitis. The Journal of Investigative Dermatology. 1984;**82**(1):30-34

[33] Sroka-Tomaszewska J, Trzeciak M. Molecular mechanisms of atopic dermatitis pathogenesis. International Journal of Molecular Sciences. 16 Apr 2021;**22**(8):4130

[34] Margolis DJ, Mitra N, Hoffstad OJ, Kim BS, Monos DS, Phillips EJ. Association of KIR genes and MHC class I ligands with atopic dermatitis. Journal of Immunology. 2021;**207**(6):1522-1529

[35] Gentle NL, Loubser S, Paximadis M, Puren A, Tiemessen CT. Killer-cell immunoglobulin-like receptor (KIR) and human leukocyte antigen (HLA) class I genetic diversity in four South African populations. Human Immunology. 2017;**78**(7-8):503-509

[36] Blokhuis JH, Hilton HG, Guethlein LA, Norman PJ, Nemat-Gorgani N, Nakimuli A, et al. KIR2DS5 allotypes that recognize the C2 epitope of HLA-C are common among Africans and absent from Europeans. Immunity, Inflammation and Disease. 2017;**5**(4):461-468

[37] Gwozdowicz S, Nestorowicz K, Graczyk-Pol E, Szlendak U, Rogatko-Koros M, Mika-Witkowska R, et al. KIR specificity and avidity of standard and unusual C1, C2, Bw4, Bw6 and A3/11 amino acid motifs at entire HLA:KIR interface between NK and target cells, the functional and evolutionary classification of HLA class I molecules. International Journal of Immunogenetics. 2019;**46**(4):217-231

[38] Kiessling R, Klein E, Wigzell H. "Natural" killer cells in the mouse. I. Cytotoxic cells with specificity for mouse Moloney leukemia cells. Specificity and distribution according to genotype. European Journal of Immunology. 1975;**5**(2):112-117

[39] Zhang L, Liu M, Yang S, Wang J, Feng X, Han Z. Natural killer cells: Of-the-shelf cytotherapy for cancer immunosurveillance. American Journal of Cancer Research. 2021;**11**(4):1770-1791

[40] Liu M, Meng Y, Zhang L, Han Z, Feng X. High-efficient generation of natural killer cells from peripheral blood with preferable cell vitality and enhanced cytotoxicity by combination of IL-2, IL-15 and IL-18. Biochemical and Biophysical Research Communications. 2021;**534**:149-156

[41] Christodoulou I, Ho WJ, Marple A, Ravich JW, Tam A, Rahnama R, et al. Engineering CAR-NK cells to secrete IL-15 sustains their anti-AML functionality but is associated with systemic toxicities. Journal for Immunotherapy of Cancer. Dec 2021;**9**(12):e003894

[42] Albinger N, Pfeifer R, Nitsche M, Mertlitz S, Campe J, Stein K, et al. Primary CD33-targeting CAR-NK cells for the treatment of acute myeloid leukemia. Blood Cancer Journal. 2022;**12**(4):61

[43] Galon J, Angell HK, Bedognetti D, Marincola FM. The continuum of cancer immunosurveillance: Prognostic, predictive, and mechanistic signatures. Immunity. 2013;**39**(1):11-26

[44] Kennedy LB, Salama AKS. A review of cancer immunotherapy toxicity. CA: A Cancer Journal for Clinicians. 2020;**70**(2):86-104

[45] Vivier E. What is natural in natural killer cells? Immunology Letters. 2006;**107**(1):1-7

[46] Xia J, Minamino S, Kuwabara K. CAR-expressing NK cells for cancer therapy: A new hope. Bioscience Trends. 2020;**14**(5):354-359

[47] Cummins KD, Gill S. Chimeric antigen receptor T-cell therapy for acute myeloid leukemia: how close to reality? Haematologica. 2019;**104**(7):1302-1308

[48] Klingemann H. Are natural killer cells superior CAR drivers? Oncoimmunology. 2014;**3**:e28147

[49] Berrien-Elliott MM, Cashen AF, Cubitt CC, Neal CC, Wong P, Wagner JA, et al. Multidimensional analyses of donor memory-like NK cells reveal new associations with response after adoptive immunotherapy for Leukemia. Cancer Discovery. 2020;**10**(12):1854-1871

[50] Zhang L, Meng Y, Feng X, Han Z. CAR-NK cells for cancer immunotherapy: From bench to bedside. Biomarker Research. 2022;**10**(1):12

[51] Tang X, Yang L, Li Z, Nalin AP, Dai H, Xu T, et al. First-in-man clinical trial of CAR NK-92 cells: Safety test of CD33-CAR NK-92 cells in patients with relapsed and refractory acute myeloid leukemia. American Journal of Cancer Research. 2018;**8**(6):1083-1089

[52] Somanchi SS, Senyukov VV, Denman CJ, Lee DA. Expansion, purification, and functional assessment of human peripheral blood NK cells. JoVE- Journal of Visualized Experiments. 2 Feb 2011;(48):2540

[53] Xie G, Dong H, Liang Y, Ham JD, Rizwan R, Chen J. CAR-NK cells: A promising cellular immunotherapy for cancer. eBioMedicine. 2020;**59**:102975

[54] Deniz G, van de Veen W, Akdis M. Natural killer cells in patients with allergic diseases. The Journal of Allergy and Clinical Immunology. 2013;**132**(3):527-535

[55] Gao H, Liu M, Zhang Y, Zhang L, Xie B. Multifaceted characterization of the biological and transcriptomic signatures of natural killer cells derived from cord blood and placental blood. Cancer Cell International. 2022;**22**(1):291

[56] Mack MR, Brestoff JR, Berrien-Elliott MM, Trier AM, Yang TB, McCullen M, et al. Blood natural killer cell deficiency reveals an immunotherapy strategy for atopic dermatitis. Science Translational Medicine. 26 Feb 2020;**12**(532):eaay1005

[57] Hayashi K, Kusakabe KT, Sugimoto S, Wakitani S, Sugi S, Kuniyoshi N, et al. Influence of atopic dermatitis on reproduction and uterine natural killer cells. The Journal of Veterinary Medical Science. 2014;**76**(6):913-916

[58] Ogg G. Natural killer cells get under your skin. Science Translational Medicine. 26 Feb 2020;**12**(532):eaba9181

[59] Alkon N, Bauer WM, Krausgruber T, Goh I, Griss J, Nguyen V, et al. Single-cell analysis reveals innate lymphoid cell lineage infidelity in atopic dermatitis. The Journal of Allergy and Clinical Immunology. 2022;**149**(2):624-639

[60] Min KY, Koo J, Noh G, Lee D, Jo MG, Lee JE, et al. CD1d(hi)PD-L1(hi) CD27(+) regulatory natural killer subset suppresses atopic dermatitis. Frontiers in Immunology. 2021;**12**:752888

Chapter 3

Leveraging Disease-Based Community Data to Provide Insights into Current Atopic Dermatitis Treatments

Ewa J. Kleczyk, Julie Mallory Crawford and Laura Dalfonso

Abstract

This chapter discusses the current landscape of Atopic Dermatitis treatment pathways and management of disease progression. Data leveraged for these types of analyses can come from disease-based communities, otherwise known as patient registries. Disease-based communities can work with participating healthcare institutions and enroll qualified patients to aid understanding of the population and sub-cohorts' characteristics, as well as therapy protocols and regimens, time to and on therapy, discontinuation trends and reasons, and healthcare outcomes. Since the data collection includes Electronic Healthcare Records (EHRs) with the ability to append patient reported outcome questionnaires, as well as any other data sources relevant to the condition being studied, the resulting datasets provide in-depth insights on the patient population and their treatment pathways. Treating physicians are the Principal Investigators, managing and monitoring the patients' progression and treatment. The reader is able, as a result, to learn the current preferred treatment pathways in treating Atopic Dermatitis, management of disease progression, as well as understand the underlying patient characteristics and historical medical information that drive the selection of therapies.

Keywords: atopic dermatitis, AD treatments, disease-based communities, patient registries, patient data processing

1. Introduction

Natural history studies and studies initiated to fulfill regulatory authority post-marketing requirements and post-marketing commitments are designed to mitigate medical and clinical knowledge gaps. However, both types of studies can be costly, slow to enroll, and inefficient in their design, as they usually are focused on a single subpopulation and may be obsolete, if or when they are completed. In contrast, using real-world data (RWD) to develop the body of evidence for disease natural history and to provide additional safety and effectiveness information needed by post-regulatory decision makers can expedite access to enhanced insights, and benefit new therapies for a broad range of patients [1]. Thus, innovative methods to acquire RWD that rapidly inform clinicians, patients, regulatory agencies, and payers are needed.

Autoimmune diseases are a broad family of immune-mediated and inflammatory diseases, which are chronic and multi-systemic. Despite being life-long in nature, in many cases, disease progression can be slowed or prevented. Unfortunately, in some instances, treatment is ineffective, and the disease is ultimately irreversible, debilitating and potentially, even life ending. According to the National Institutes of Health, over 23 million Americans have an autoimmune disease [2]. More than 1 million adults are estimated to have rheumatoid arthritis (RA); 7.5 million have psoriasis (PsO); 204,000 have systemic lupus erythematosus (SLE); 53,000–248,000 are diagnosed with Sjogren's Syndrome (SS); between 330,000 to 1.6 million are estimated to have ankylosing spondylitis (AS); and from 330,000 to 660,000 have psoriatic arthritis (PsA) [3–9].

Immune-mediated inflammatory skin conditions (IMISCs) are a subset of autoimmune diseases, and include atopic dermatitis (AD), PsO, hidradenitis suppurativa (HS), vitiligo, alopecia areata (AA), chronic spontaneous urticaria (CSU), and dermatomyositis. These are chronic, inflammatory disorders affecting the skin and appendages. They constitute a substantial financial burden on the U.S. health care system [10] and are among the greatest contributors to the burden of skin disease worldwide [11].

The etiologies of IMISCs are still being elucidated and are thought to be related to a combination of factors, including genetic susceptibility, social and environmental exposures, immune abnormalities, and skin barrier aberrations. IMISCs can affect individuals of all ages and typically wax and wane over time, with asymptomatic periods that may span days to decades. For example, AD often presents early in childhood with intense itching and recurrent eczematous skin lesions. Originally regarded as a childhood disorder mediated by a T-helper-2 dominated inflammatory response. AD is now recognized as a lifelong disposition with variable clinical manifestations [12]. Defects of the epidermal barrier, immune dysregulation, and environmental factors are thought to affect disease expression over time [13].

Selection of therapies for IMISCs is based upon various characteristics, including patient preferences, location and type of involvement, and risk factors for more severe disease. The pharmacologic options for management of IMISCs have expanded greatly over the past 15 years, based on growing knowledge of the immune pathways involved, with further expansion expected over the next decade. Prior to 2003, when the first biologic agents were FDA approved for the treatment of psoriasis, medical therapies had consisted of topical emollients and corticosteroids, phototherapy, and non-specific immunosuppressive treatments such as methotrexate and cyclosporine. Since that time, treatment patterns have shifted toward more targeted therapies [12, 13].

This chapter is focused primarily on atopic dermatitis (AD) and presents the current market condition, treatment pathways, and changing treatment environment. In the United States, the reported prevalence of AD in adults is 5% and that for children ranges from 10 to 20% [14, 15]. Symptoms of AD include pruritis, xerosis, lichenification, and sleep disturbance. In infants and young children, skin findings typically occur on the scalp, face, and extensor surfaces of the extremities. Older children and adults typically have involvement of the flexor surfaces, neck, wrists and ankles [16].

Risk factors for the development of AD include filaggrin gene mutations and family history of atopic or allergic disease [17]. Flares of AD are triggered by irritants, such as soaps, and allergens, such as food allergies. Comorbid diseases that are associated with AD include asthma, attention-deficit hyperactivity disorders (ADHD) and autism spectrum disorder (ASD) [18].

There are several challenges associated with drug discovery in autoimmune diseases, including the limited understanding of the biology and natural-history of each specific disease, as well as the appropriate targets for disease-modifying therapies. This is further complicated by a lack of early diagnosis. It has been shown that early intervention in autoimmune disease generally leads to better outcomes and that aggressive treatments can often halt disease progression. The concept of treat-to-target to track progress toward a predefined outcome and adjust dosing, accordingly, has also been a growing influence on autoimmune disease treatment for more than a decade, yet in some cases is not recommended.

Many of the same categories of medicinal treatment are used across the autoimmune diseases, including dermatological conditions, another indicator of a possible common etiology. Treatments frequently assessed in studies include:

- NSAIDs, non-steroidal anti-inflammatory drugs (e.g., acetaminophen and meloxicam)
- Corticosteroids (CCS, e.g., prednisone and methylprednisolone)
- Disease Modifying Anti-Rheumatic Drugs (DMARD)
    - Immunosuppressants and conventional synthetics (csDMARD): Azathioprine, Cyclosporine, Cyclophosphamide, Hydroxychloroquine (anti-malarial), Leflunomide, Methotrexate, Mycophenolate mofetil, Sulfasalazine, Calcineurin inhibitors
    - Biologic inhibitors (bDMARD): IL-17, IL-23, B-Cell, CTLA4, TNF, BLyS/BAFF
    - Targeted Small Molecules (tsDMARD): Janus kinase inhibitors, PDE-4 inhibitors
- Other IMISC therapies: topical emollients, phototherapy

Due to the prevalence of autoimmune diseases, there is an increasing need to develop multiple pathways that unlock the potential of real-world data (RWD) and real-world evidence (RWE) to improve patient outcomes and inform clinical trial design, especially in underserved patient populations. The current approach to healthcare is informed mostly by clinical trials with sample sizes in the hundreds or few thousands, which limits generalizability to broader patient populations and can be impractical due to costs and feasibility. In 2020, FDA issued a draft guidance identifying that there are a number of underserved patient groups (e.g., ethnic minorities, women, elderly, those at the extremes of weight range, individuals with organ dysfunction, those with malignancies or certain infections such as HIV, and children) who are routinely excluded from trials without sufficient clinical or scientific justification [19]. The exclusionary nature of our current healthcare system limits the generalizability of the study results to the wider population. Furthermore, in 2022, FDA released another draft guidance, encouraging sponsors of drug trials to outline a Diversity Plan as part of their submissions. In particular, when data suggest a difference in performance of the product based on factors related to race or ethnicity, the Diversity Plan should specify a roadmap for informing safety and effectiveness for each relevant population [20].

The rapid integration of Electronic Health Records (EHRs) has made longitudinal clinical data available for research, making real-world data (RWD) and the real-world evidence (RWE) derived from them an increasingly important tool in modern healthcare systems [21]. By aggregating real-world health and disease information from tens of thousands to hundreds of thousands or more diverse patients via EHR systems, the scale and scope of studies of a wide range of diseases, both common and rare, are improved by adding statistical power to detect associations between various complex factors and a wide variety of outcomes. The increasing utilization of RWD is further enhanced by the growing sophistication of epidemiologic and statistical methods that can facilitate principled learning. These include the development and refinement of causal inference methods, which permit the control of large numbers of covariates, and extend naturally to complex, longitudinal data, which allow (under certain assumptions) for the estimation of the effects of different care pathways for chronic disease [22–31]. Recent guidance issued by the FDA regarding the utilization of RWE to facilitate drug development underscores the importance of these data sources [32].

As a result of the importance of understanding the autoimmune diseases, this chapter leverages RWD in the form of disease-based communities, otherwise known as patient registries, and presents the current market landscape for AD and available treatment options.

2. A disease-based community's (patient registry) overview

In a disease-based community, otherwise known as a patient registry, patient level data is collected for the purpose of starting an observational research study. The objective of the community is to present a comprehensive review of outcomes for patients with specific diseases. The registry includes patients being managed for select diseases in usual clinical practice in the United States to address important clinical questions, regarding the management of these diseases by collecting and analyzing data from patients at a variety of academic medical centers and community medical practices. Practice patterns often vary by practice type, location, and the population treated, so the ability to study patients based on the specifics of their clinic type is useful. The study is designed to develop a robust database of real-world data regarding the natural history and health outcomes related to the management of diseases of diverse etiologies. Some examples of disease registries are shown in **Figure 1**. In the example below, the dermatology community includes a subset of patients with AD [33].

The dermatology disease-based community enrolls patients from dermatology and allergy clinics that manage various dermatologic diseases, including AD, AA, HS, and CSU. Patients with AD are the primary focus of this chapter. The patients participating in a dermatology registry provide consent for their Electronic Health Records (EHRs) to be shared for research purposes. The data includes EHR for up to the prior 3 years retrospectively from the date of patient consent as well as prospective records. Prospective medical record collection continues for up to 15 years or until a study completion/exit criterion is met. The submitted records (structured and unstructured data) include but are not limited to inpatient and outpatient notes, pharmacy records, laboratory data, radiographic and procedure reports, histology reports, and all prior

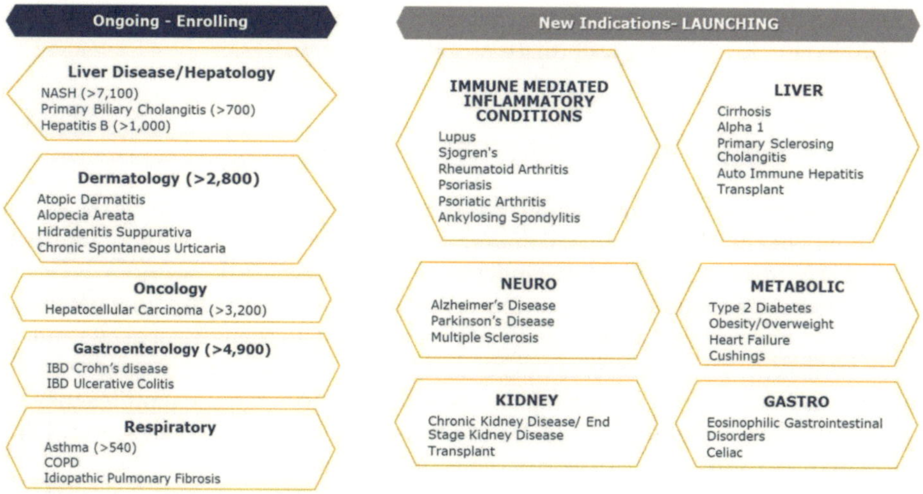

Figure 1.
Examples of currently available and upcoming disease-based communities.

clinical details specific to screening methods, diagnostic evaluation, and treatment regimens for the studied conditions, along with associated comorbid conditions and complications [33].

The medical records include, but are not limited to [33]:

- clinic notes/encounters and telephone contact notes/reports
- laboratory, radiographic, imaging, or other reports
- medication lists/pharmacy reports
- hospitalization records
- procedures

Records include all prior clinical details specific to screening methods, diagnostic evaluation, and treatment regimens of the respective dermatologic disease, including reasons for premature discontinuation of any therapies and treatment response [33].

Patients can also consent to participate in Patient Reported Outcomes (PRO) surveys and health-related questionnaires. Patients may also be invited to optionally provide periodic biospecimens. Patients can be enrolled at a regularly scheduled clinic visit or consented remotely as is permissible by each site's IRB [33].

Utilizing this approach for data collection provides an efficient solution to collect information about critical populations from real-world practice, often underrepresented in clinical trials and disadvantaged in the US healthcare system. The concept is to avoid influencing practice patterns, instead capturing the standard of care at the given sites. The data also informs natural history studies and may provide a post-marketing safety and effectiveness surveillance platform that is otherwise impracticable from consented cohorts. It may also provide a platform from which to identify deficiencies in care, determine best practices, and evaluate patient and health outcomes in special subpopulations with the potential to improve the overall quality of care for patients with autoimmune diseases [33].

For the purpose of the chapter, the following AD diagnosis codes are leveraged: L20-L20.9; H01.131-139 atopic dermatitis/eczema, various.

3. Patient reported outcomes for atopic dermatitis

A patient-reported outcome (PRO) has been defined as "Any report of the status of a patient's health condition that comes directly from the patient, without interpretation of the patient's response by a clinician or anyone else" [34].

Self-reported patient health measures collect information directly from patients/caregivers to measure physical, mental, and social health in their disease state and during treatment. These measures can be used to help clinicians better understand how various treatments affect what patients are able to do and the symptoms they experience beyond what is typically derived from traditional clinical measures. The information can also be used to help patients make informed decisions about their healthcare and treatment options. Both the PROMIS initiative (Patient-Reported Outcome Measurement Information System) from the NIH and PCORI (Patient Centered-Outcomes Research Institute) have highlighted the need to implement patient centered measures into health care delivery. As a result, many healthcare organizations are implementing patient reported outcomes instruments as part of the standard patient intake for clinical visits and management [35].

In evaluating Atopic Dermatitis, outcomes data are sometimes collected at clinical visits to measure response, or lack of response to treatment, and can sometimes be reflected in routine clinical documentation. Types of information collected can include data about itch, location, itch frequency and severity and sleep disturbance. Other disease-specific PROs that are not part of routine clinical care may be collected through additional questionnaires at the start of the study and at regular follow up intervals. These may also include data on quality of life, neuropsychiatric (depression and anxiety) measures, how the condition may or may not impair work function, etc., as these are not only important to understanding the condition but can also sometimes affect treatment outcomes. There are many PROs available for AD, including the examples below [35].

Data on diagnosis can be collected through the U.K. Working Party Criteria (UKWPC) [36, 37], while data related to itch is captured through the Patient Oriented Eczema Measure (POEM) [38], which has been previously used in treatment trials for Atopic Dermatitis and other inflammatory skin disease states. The Patient-Oriented-SCORing Atopic Dermatitis (PO-SCORAD) [39] captures data related to severity. The Atopic Dermatitis Control Tool, (ADCT) [40] data related to itch, sleep, and quality of life. Itch, pain, and sleep can also be assessed by numeric rating scales. Quality of life, work impairment, and anxiety and depression can be assessed using the Dermatology Life Quality Index (DLQI) [41], Work Productivity and Impairment Questionnaire (WAPI) [42], or the PROMIS "PIQ" Short Forms, respectively [42].

The Children's Dermatology Life Quality Index (CDLQI) [43] and the Infants Dermatitis Quality of Life Index (IDQOL) [44] are validated tools that assess disease activity in infants, children, and adolescents. The PROMIS Pediatric Scales assess anxious and depressive symptoms in children, as well as those related to sleep and itch [44].

In addition to patient reported outcome measures, Clinician Reported Outcomes (ClinROs) are an important data point in all disease areas. In AD, ClinROs are particularly important, given the scarcity of detail in clinician notes. Two of the most widely used ClinROsin AD include the Eczema Area and Severity Index (EASI) and the validated Investigator Global Assessment for Atopic Dermatitis (vIGA-AD) [45]. The EASI evaluates the severity of disease using an area score in each body region. The vIGA looks at overall severity of AD at the time of the exam. At times, clinicians also estimate a body surface area (BSA), the percent of skin affected by AD at the time of the exam [45].

4. Patient data processing overview

The patient registry provides a small-footprint data acquisition engine to process the EHR source (structured and unstructured data) of patients and export it from sites. The process typically is executed within the site firewall but can also be performed under secure protocols at managing organization or even at a mutually agreed Trusted Third Party (TTP) [33].

The data is standardized, pre-processed, and packaged behind the site firewall before being securely transmitted to the technical platform. The preprocessing and standardization steps allow for "at source" validation of the data elements extracted from the upstream system. Patient data from the sites is transmitted at frequent fixed intervals (weekly/monthly) and each site has a deterministic update schedule so that missing data receipts can be flagged [33].

This approach provides an EHR-agnostic strategy and utilizes a standard extract/report format most frequently available for the site's EHR system, such as the Fast Healthcare Interoperability Resources (FHIR) standard. Such standard data extract formats will reduce ongoing support required by the sites technical team [33].

5. Methodology overview

Descriptive summaries are the basis of reporting used to support any insights derived in this chapter.

Numeric measures, including shifts from baseline, if possible, are summarized with the available number of patients (n), median, minimum, and maximum values. The mean, standard deviation, standard error, quartiles, inter quartile range, and number of missing observations may optionally be reported. Applicable figures include histograms, box plots, scatter plots, mean ± standard deviations, and mean ± standard errors.

Categorical descriptive measures are summarized with counts and percentages. The denominator in fixed category variables will be the number of patients with an observed result. The denominator for medication or defined event summaries represents all patients who could have had an observation. Defined events may also include the total number of events or the events per period. Cumulative event rates may be calculated using Kaplan-Meier methods.

6. Atopic dermatitis current market landscape overview

Through a series of quarterly reported summary statistics and insights, a snapshot of the AD patient registry is published every 3 months over the course of the registry. Patients included in the study started enrolling in January 2019 and have data from up to 3 years prior to that date, so the AD dataset captures several years of longitudinal data, including any events available post diagnosis. The below write up summarizes key insights from the currently available AD data.

In the Dermatology disease-based community cohort, there are currently 3559 participants enrolled in the US and Canada, of whom 2774 are included in the atopic dermatitis cohort. Of those, 2755 (99%) are included in this chapter market assessment. There are 53 active sites and 7 closed sites. The participants in this report represent 50 sites in the US and Canada; 25 of these sites are community and 25 are academic. A well-balanced sample of sites is important in ensuring unbiased insights.

One goal of registry studies is to be more representative of diverse populations than randomized clinical trials are able to be. Demographic summary statistics present the sex and racial/ethnic breakdown of the cohort. For example, there are 1514 female participants (55%) and 1241 male participants (45%). 1495 participants represent adults in the sample. There are 1428 White (52%), 346 (13%) African American, 15 (0.5%) American Indian or Alaskan Native, 18 (1%) Native Hawaiian or Other Pacific Islander, and 244 (9%) Asian participants. There are 19% Hispanics of any race in the cohort. The sex and racial/ethnic breakdown present similar ratios as noted in other registry studies [14, 15]. Systematic reviews of randomized clinical trials have shown a lag in terms of transparency of race and ethnicity reporting in dermatology studies; this has started to shift [46].

In addition, therapies taken at any time are reported by age group and organized by systemic therapy, topical therapy, and phototherapy. The recently approved JAK inhibitor and monoclonal antibody therapies, for instance, are tracked over time; there is great interest in observing the uptake of these therapies in the registry to understand the changing trends in treatments. Over time, sequencing of therapies will also be followed and reported. In addition, trends in topical therapy use are documented. Some therapies, like corticosteroids, are reported in multiple sections, as their route of administration includes both a systemic and topical option.

In this cohort, which is enriched by patients with moderate-to-severe disease, both systemic and topical therapies are widely prescribed. For the systemic therapies, antihistamines—often available over the counter—are often used, with hydroxyzine being the most frequently dosed treatment. Hydroxyzine is the only first-generation antihistamine that is recommended for AD. Monoclonal antibodies such as dupilumab are also used in this patient population [47]. Adults have a higher share of dupilumab use when compared to pediatric patients, which is likely due to the earlier approval date for adults. More recently, several other systemic biologic therapies have gained approval in the United States and other parts of the world. These therapies include tralokinumab, which is another monoclonal antibody, and upadacitinib, abrocitinib, and baricitinib, which are janus-kinase inhibitors (JAK-inhibitors). With regard to topical therapies, crisaborole (a phosphodiase-4 inhibitor) and ruxolitinib (another JAK-inhibitor) are creams that are approved for mild to moderate patients with AD. In addition, other topical therapies include calcineurin inhibitors and topical antibiotics. Finally, the vast majority of patients take either systemic or topical corticosteroids. Please note that the share of drug utilization often varies by the patient segment and the corresponding disease severity. As additional patient data is collected, more in-depth trends will be reported, including as noted above sequencing of treatments.

Most often prescribed concomitant therapies include treatments for health issues related to the respiratory system, alimentary track and metabolism, nervous system, and cardiovascular system. AD patients also often experience other types of allergic diagnoses from allergies to grass, weed and tree pollen, dust mice, food such as milk, nuts, and gluten to allergies to pets. While there are several different types of allergies, many of them are only experienced by a small percent of patients. As noted in other articles, the findings confirm previously found insights that comorbid diseases that are associated with AD include asthma and depression, but not noted in this analysis, attention-deficit hyperactivity disorders (ADHD) and autism spectrum disorder (ASD) have also been found to be associated [18].

Another important statistic shows the ClinRO responses at the time of the quarterly report (**Figure 2**). It is important to note the distribution of vIGA-AD severity score, which includes patients with clear or almost clear skin alongside patients with more severe categories of AD. Interestingly, this measure does not account for the type of therapy the patient was taking at the time of the clinician assessment. For example, a patient on dupilumab, who previously had severe AD, but is now well-controlled on therapy, might be reported to have a clear vIGA-AD score. In analyses, factors like this can be accounted for and worked into other reports. The summary results are intended to be idea-generating, and to encourage thoughts for analyses and publications on the registry data.

As shown in **Figure 2**, based on the validated Investigator Global Assessment for Atopic Dermatitis (vIGA-ADTM) at study enrollment, 216 (8%) were rated as clear, 381 (14%) as almost clear, 738 (27%) as mild, 1046 (38%) as moderate and 364 (13%) as severe.

It is important to note that while initially open to all patients being managed for AD, the AD patient enrollment is currently limited to patients who met the following targeted criteria: those with a vIGA score of moderate or severe at the time of enrollment, those who are currently on a biologic therapy or one of the following systemic treatments (methotrexate, cyclosporine, mycophenolate mofetil, novel biologics/JAK inhibitors and oral steroids) and those with a history of moderate or severe chronic

	Age Group			
Characteristic	Pediatric[3] (N=977)	Adolescent[4] (N=283)	Adult[5] (N=1495)	All participants (N=2755)
vIGA-AD Score, n (%)				
n	977	283	1495	2755
Clear	50 (5.1%)	16 (5.7%)	150 (10.0%)	216 (7.8%)
Almost clear	150 (15.4%)	31 (11.0%)	200 (13.4%)	381 (13.8%)
Mild	256 (26.2%)	75 (26.5%)	407 (27.2%)	738 (26.8%)
Moderate	372 (38.1%)	110 (38.9%)	564 (37.7%)	1046 (38.0%)
Severe	145 (14.8%)	51 (18.0%)	168 (11.2%)	364 (13.2%)
Not Reported	4 (0.4%)	0 (0.0%)	6 (0.4%)	10 (0.4%)
Total BSA				
Median (n)	9 (973)	8 (283)	5 (1489)	7 (2745)
Min - Max	0 - 100	0 - 95	0 - 100	0 - 100
Q1 - Q3 (IQR)	4 - 25	3 - 20	2 - 15	2 - 20

[1]Validated Investigator Global Assessment Scale for Atopic Dermatitis
[2]Total Body Surface Area Percent Reported
[3]Participants with age <=12
[4]Participants with age 13 to 17
[5]Participants with age >17

Figure 2.
vIGA-AD[1] and total BSA[2] status at enrollment by participant type.

AD, as supported by documentation in the available retrospective medical records. The reason for these targeted criteria is to enhance the population of patients who are eligible to receive treatment with the newer systemic therapies entering the market. Information on their performance in the real world is critical.

There is also great interest in seeing many of the summary statistics broken out by age group. Not only are different age groups affected by AD in unique ways, but therapies are also approved for different age groups at different times. So, for example, a new therapy might be available for adults prior to its label extending to adolescent or pediatric patients.

Finally, there is also interest in seeing summary statistics broken out by the site setting. In a well-balanced registry, patients will come from both community and academic sites. For this reporting period includes 1495 adult participants; 506 (31%) of the adult participants are enrolled at academic study sites and 989 (66%) are enrolled at community sites. This summary report includes 1260 pediatric patients; 635 (50%) of the pediatric participants are enrolled at academic study sites and 625 (50%) are enrolled at community sites.

7. Conclusions

This chapter introduced the concept of disease-based communities, otherwise known as patient registries and presented the AD market assessment based on to date available data to date. Patient registries are an important collection model of medical records that allow for receiving in-depth insights related to the patient diagnoses and treatment pathways as well as overall patient journey. The data provides a variety of data elements, such as clinic notes, laboratory, radiographic, imaging reports, prescribed medication lists, and diagnostic procedures and results. The level of granularity of the data is not always found in the healthcare claims, remittance, pharmacy adjudicated information, and primary market research datasets. The information can aid the understanding of patient outcomes, disease progression, and best pathways for treatment application, and fill in missing gaps from the other data sources. The deeper understanding of the AD diagnostic and treatment patterns, as a result, can help deploy strategies to optimize the care process, ultimately improving patient quality of life and final outcomes.

The overall disease-based community insights present that most patients' diagnoses with AD are treated with at least a topical drug application, but often also systemic therapies such as antihistamines, monoclonal antibodies, and JAK-inhibitors. In addition, a small percent of patients has other allergies and are treated for a variety of comorbid conditions such as respiratory and cardiovascular diseases. Female patients represent a slightly higher percentage of AD patients in this registry, while from race/ethnic breakdown, 'White' patients represent half of the studied sample.

As noted earlier, due to still relatively small sample size in the patient registry, the level of insights presented in this chapter is limited. Future research will include reporting trends in combinations of therapies, reasons for discontinuing therapies, response to treatment over time, subsets of the population that respond to various therapies, PROs, and ClinROs over time and in relation to therapy starts.

Furthermore, with the larger sample, ability for inferential analysis vs. just descriptive statistics reporting will be available to provide additional insights into the data elements, impacting the diagnoses, disease progressions, and types of treatment prescribed. Survival analytics and adherence analytics represent examples of analytics that could be applied to the larger dataset. Other examples of analytics include predictive analytics, next best action analytics, and other marketing and management sciences analyses.

Acknowledgements

Authors would like to thank Keith Knapp, PhD, Target RWE, Durham, NC, USA for his contribution to this book chapter.

Funding

Authors work for Target RWE organization.

Conflict of interest

The authors declare no conflict of interest.

Nomenclature

AA	Alopecia Areata
AD	Atopic Dermatitis
ADCT	Atopic Dermatitis Control Tool
ADHD	Attention-Deficit Hyperactivity Disorders
ASD	Autism Spectrum Disorder
AS	Ankylosing Spondylitis
BSA	Body Area Surface
CDLQI	Children's Dermatology Life Quality Index
ClinRO	Clinician Reported Outcomes
CSU	Chronic Spontaneous Urticaria
DLQI	Dermatology Life Quality Index
EHR	Electronic Healthcare Records
FDA	U. S. Food and Drug Administration
FHIR	Fast Healthcare Interoperability Resources
HS	Hidradenitis Suppurativa
IDQOL	Infants Dermatitis Quality of Life Index
IMISCs	Immune-Mediated Inflammatory Skin Conditions
POEM	Patient Oriented Eczema Measure
PO-SCORAD	Patient-Oriented-SCORing Atopic Dermatitis
PRO	Patient Reported Outcomes
PROMIS	"PIQ" Short Forms
PsO	Psoriasis
RA	Rheumatoid Arthritis
RWD	Real-World Data
RWE	Real-World Evidence
SLE	Systemic Lupus Erythematosus

SS	Sjogren's Syndrome
TTP	Trusted Third Party
UKWPC	U.K. Working Party Criteria
vIGA	Validated Investigator Global Assessment
WAPI	Work Productivity and Impairment Questionnaire

Author details

Ewa J. Kleczyk[1,2*], Julie Mallory Crawford[1] and Laura Dalfonso[1]

1 Target RWE, Durham, NC, USA

2 The University of Maine, Orono, ME, USA

*Address all correspondence to: ekleczyk@targetrwe.com

References

[1] Abuabara K, Silverberg JI, Simpson EL, Paller AS, Eichenfield LF, Bissonnette R, et al. International observational atopic dermatitis cohort to follow natural history and treatment course: TARGET-DERM AD study design and rationale. BMJ Open. 2020;**10**(11):e039928. DOI: 10.1136/bmjopen-2020-039928. PMID: 33247014; PMCID: PMC7703415

[2] NIH Autoimmune Diseases Coordinating Committee: Autoimmune Diseases Research Plan, 2005. Available from: https://www.niaid.nih.gov/sites/default/files/adccfinal.pdf [Accessed: October 3, 2022]

[3] Hunter TM, Boytsov NN, Zhang X, et al. Prevalence of rheumatoid arthritis in the United States adult population in healthcare claims databases, 2004-2014. Rheumatology International. 2017;**37**:1551-1557

[4] Rachakonda TD, Schupp CW, Armstrong AW. Psoriasis prevalence among adults in the United States. Journal of the American Academy of Dermatology. 2014;**70**(3):512-516

[5] Armstrong AW, Mehta MD, Schupp CW, Gondo GC, Bell SJ, Griffiths CEM. Psoriasis prevalence in adults in the United States. JAMA Dermatology. 2021;**157**(8):940-946

[6] Izmirly PM, Parton H, Wang L, McCune WJ, Lim SS, Drenkard C, et al. Prevalence of systemic lupus erythematosus in the United States: Estimates from a meta-analysis of the centers for disease control and prevention national lupus registries. Arthritis & Rhematology. 2021;**73**(6):991-996

[7] Maciel G, Crowson CS, Matteson EL, Cornec D. Prevalence of primary Sjögren's syndrome in a US population-based cohort. Arthritis Care and Research (Hoboken). 2017;**69**(10):1612-1616

[8] Taurog JD, Chhabra A, Colbert RA. Ankylosing spondylitis and axial Spondyloarthritis. The New England Journal of Medicine. 2016;**374**(26):2563-2574

[9] Saalfeld W, Mixon AM, Zelie J, Lydon EJ. Differentiating psoriatic arthritis from osteoarthritis and rheumatoid arthritis: A narrative review and guide for advanced practice providers. Rheumatology and Therapy. 2021;**8**(4):1493-1517

[10] Lim HW, Collins SAB, Resneck JS Jr, Bolognia JL, Hodge JA, Rohrer TA, et al. The burden of skin disease in the United States. Journal of the American Academy of Dermatology. 2017;**76**(5):958-972.e2

[11] Hay RJ, Johns NE, Williams HC, Bolliger IW, Dellavalle RP, Margolis DJ, et al. The global burden of skin disease in 2010: An analysis of the prevalence and impact of skin conditions. The Journal of Investigative Dermatology. 2014;**134**(6):1527-1534

[12] Weidinger S, Novak N. Atopic dermatitis. Lancet. 2016;**387**(10023):1109-1122

[13] Leung DY, Guttman-Yassky E. Deciphering the complexities of atopic dermatitis: Shifting paradigms in treatment approaches. The Journal of Allergy and Clinical Immunology. 2014;**134**(4):769-779

[14] Barbarot S, Auziere S, Gadkari A, Girolomoni G, Puig L, Simpson EL, et al. Epidemiology of atopic dermatitis

in adults: Results from an international survey. Allergy. 2018;**73**(6):1284-1293. DOI: 10.1111/all.13401

[15] Eichenfield et al. Atopic Dermatitis: Epidemiology and Pathogenesis Update. Seminars in cutaneous medicine and surgery. Elsevier Science; 2012;**31**:S3-S5

[16] McAleer MA, O'Regan GM, et al. Atopic dermatitis. In: Bolognia JL et al., editors. Dermatology. 4th ed. Vol. 208. China: Elsevier; 2018. p. 27

[17] Simpson et al. Update on epidemiology, diagnosis, and disease course of atopic dermatitis. Seminars in Cutaneous Medicine and Surgery. 2016;**35**:S84-S88. DOI: 10.12788/j.sder.2016.041

[18] Leung DYM et al. New insights into atopic dermatitis. Journal of Clinical Investigation. 2004;**113**(5):651-657

[19] U.S. Department of Health and Human Services, Food and Drug Administration et al. Enhancing the Diversity of Clinical Trial Populations—Eligibility Criteria, Enrollment Practices, and Trials Designs. Guidance for Industry. Rockville, MD: Food and Drug Administration; 2020. Available from: https://www.fda.gov/media/127212/download. [Accessed: October 3, 2022]

[20] U.S. Department of Health and Human Services, Food and Drug Administration et al. FDA Takes Important Steps to Increase Racial and Ethnic Diversity in Clinical Trials. Guidance for Industry. Rockville, MD: Food and Drug Administration; 2022. Available from: https://www.fda.gov/news-events/press-announcements/fda-takes-important-steps-increase-racial-and-ethnic-diversity-clinical-trials. [Accessed: December 11, 2022]

[21] NEJM CATALYST. Healthcare Big Data and the Promise of Value-Based Care. NEJM CATALYST: NEJM; 2018. Available from: https://catalyst.nejm.org/doi/full/10.1056/CAT.18.0290. [Accessed: January 28, 2023]

[22] Robins JM, Hernan MA, Brumback B. Marginal structural models and causal inference in epidemiology. Epidemiology. 2000;**11**:550-560

[23] An der Laan MJ, Robins JM. Unified Methods for Censored and Longitudinal Data and Causality. New York: Springer Verlag; 2002

[24] Schneeweiss S. Learning from big health care data. The New England Journal of Medicine. 2014;**370**:2161-2163

[25] Cepeda MS, Boston R, Farrar JT, Strom BL. Comparison of logistic regression versus propensity score when the number of events is low and there are multiple confounders. American Journal of Epidemiology. 2003;**158**:280-287

[26] Seeger JD, Walker AM, Williams PL, Saperia GM, Sacks FM. A propensity score-matched cohort study of the effect of statins, mainly fluvastatin, on the occurrence of acute myocardial infarction. The American Journal of Cardiology. 2003;**92**:1447-1451

[27] Seeger JD, Kurth T, Walker AM. Use of propensity score technique to account for exposure-related covariates: An example and lesson. Medical Care. 2007;**45**:S143-S148

[28] Brookhart MA, Reams D, Dluzniewski PJ, Kshirsagar A, Walsh L, Bradbury BD. Estimating the effect of preventable treatment discontinuation on health outcomes. Epidemiology. 2018;**29**:134-141

[29] Hernan MA, Lanoy E, Costagliola D, Robins JM. Comparison of dynamic treatment regimes via inverse

probability weighting. Basic & Clinical Pharmacology & Toxicology. 2006;**98**:237-242

[30] Cain LE, Saag MS, Petersen M, et al. Using observational data to emulate a randomized trial of dynamic treatment-switching strategies: An application to antiretroviral therapy. International Journal of Epidemiology. 2016;**45**:2038-2049

[31] U.S. Department of Health and Human Services Food and Drug Administration Center for Drug Evaluation and Research (CDER). Real-world data: Assessing electronic health records and medical claims data to support regulatory decision-making for drug and biological products. Guidance for Industry. 2021

[32] Mishra P, Florian J, Peter J, Vainorius M, Fried MW, Nelson DR, et al. Public–private partnership: Targeting real-world data for hepatitis C direct-acting antivirals. Gastroenterology. 2017;**153**:626-631

[33] Target RWE. Partners for the Real World. Durham, NC: Target RWE; 2022. Available from: https://www.targetrwe.com/. [Accessed: December 10, 2022]

[34] U.S. Food and Drug Administration. Patient-reported outcome measures: Use in medical product development to support labeling claims. Guidance for Industry. Rockville, MD: Food and Drug Administration. 2009;**74**(35):65132-65133. Available from: https://www.fda.gov/regulatory-information/search-fda-guidance-documents/patient-reported-outcome-measures-use-medical-product-development-support-labeling-claims. [Accessed: December 9, 2022]

[35] Target RWE. Patient Reported Outcomes—Site Starter Packet. Internal Company Marketing and Training Resources; 2022 [Accessed: December 10, 2022]

[36] Williams HC, Burney PG, Hay RJ, et al. The UK working party's diagnostic criteria for atopic dermatitis. I. Derivation of a minimum set of discriminators for atopic dermatitis. The British Journal of Dermatology. 1994;**131**:383-396

[37] Williams HC, Burney PG, Pembroke AC, et al. The UK working party's diagnostic criteria for atopic dermatitis. III. Independent hospital validation. The British Journal of Dermatology. 1994;**131**:406-416

[38] Spuls PI, Gerbens LAA, Simpson E, et al. Patient-oriented eczema measure (POEM), a core instrument to measure symptoms in clinical trials: A harmonising outcome measures for eczema (home) statement. The British Journal of Dermatology. 2017;**176**:979-984

[39] Stalder J-F, Barbarot S, Wollenberg A, et al. Patient-oriented SCORAD (PO-SCORAD): A new self-assessment scale in atopic dermatitis validated in Europe. Allergy. 2011;**66**:1114-1121

[40] Simpson E, Eckert L, Gadkari A, Mallya UG, Yang M, Nelson L, et al. Validation of the atopic dermatitis control tool (ADCT©) using a longitudinal survey of biologic-treated patients with atopic dermatitis. BMC Dermatology. 2019;**19**(1):15. DOI: 10.1186/s12895-019-0095-3

[41] Basra MKA, Fenech R, Gatt RM, et al. The dermatology life quality index 1994-2007: A comprehensive review of validation data and clinical results. The British Journal of Dermatology. 2008;**159**:997-1035

[42] Reilly MC, Zbrozek AS, Dukes EM. The validity and reproducibility of a work productivity and activity impairment instrument. PharmacoEconomics. 1993;**4**:353-365

[43] Lewis-Jones MS, Finlay AY. The children's dermatology life quality index (CDLQI): Initial validation and practical use. The British Journal of Dermatology. 1995;**132**:942-949

[44] Hanifin JM, Thurston M, Omoto M, et al. The eczema area and severity index (EASI): Assessment of reliability in atopic dermatitis. EASI Evaluator Group. Experimental Dermatology. 2001;**10**(1):11-18. DOI: 10.1034/j.1600-0625.2001.100102.x

[45] Eli Lilly and Company. Validated Investigator Global Assessment. Used with the Permission of Eli Lilly and Company under a Creative Commons Attribution-No Derivatives 4.0 international license. 2017

[46] Chen V, Akhtar S, Zheng C, Kumaresan V, Nouri K. Assessment of changes in diversity in dermatology clinical trials between 2010-2015 and 2015-2020: A systematic review. JAMA Dermatology. 2022;**158**(3):288-292. DOI: 10.1001/jamadermatol.2021.5596

[47] Nowicki R, Trzeciak M, Wilkowska A, Sokołowska-Wojdyło M, Ługowska-Umer H, Barańska-Rybak W, et al. Atopic dermatitis: Current treatment guidelines. Statement of the experts of the dermatological section, polish Society of Allergology, and the allergology section, polish Society of Dermatology. Advances in Dermatology and Allergology. 2015;**32**(4):239-249. DOI: 10.5114/pdia.2015.53319

Chapter 4

An Era of Therapeutic Evolution and Revolution: Insights into Studies on Dupilumab, Tralokinumab, Lebrikizumab, Nemolizumab, Eblasakimab, and OX40/OX40L Agents (Rocatinlimab and Amlitelimab) in Moderate-to-Severe Atopic Dermatitis

Charbel Skayem and Tu Anh Duong

Abstract

Atopic dermatitis (AD), a prevalent chronic inflammatory skin condition, presents with diverse phenotypes and endotypes. Traditional treatments have included topical corticosteroids, phototherapy, calcineurin inhibitors, and systemic immunosuppressants, the latter often necessitating frequent lab monitoring due to concerns about adverse effects. Recently, the AD treatment landscape has evolved significantly, marked by the introduction of innovative therapies. This advancement is driven by the identification of biomarkers predictive of therapeutic responses and the integration of bench research, leading to improved disease stratification and treatment selection. Emerging therapies, particularly monoclonal antibodies and targeted treatments, have shown exceptional efficacy in managing moderate-to-severe AD. This chapter focuses on clinical trials evaluating the effectiveness of these novel biologic agents other than JAK inhibitors.

Keywords: atopic dermatitis, biologics, novel treatment, dupilumab, tralokinumab, lebrikizumab, nemolizumab, eblasakimab, OX40/OX40L agents

1. Introduction

Atopic dermatitis (AD) is one the most common chronic inflammatory skin diseases, with a variety of phenotypes and endotypes. In recent decades, treatments have been based on topical corticosteroids, phototherapy, calcineurin inhibitors, and systemic immunosuppressants. However, with systemic immunosuppressant therapy, many patients require frequent laboratory monitoring and some are undertreated for concerns regarding adverse effects [1]. In the last decade, the therapeutic pipeline of AD has been enriched. As a consequence, there has been an emergence of novel and promising therapeutic perspectives. The identification of biomarkers that can have therapeutic responses as well as the integration of bench studies are the key to this translational revolution. This novel approach led to a better disease stratification and a better therapeutic selection.

New agents have been developed, including monoclonal antibodies and narrow targeting therapies, which proved to outstanding efficacy against moderate-to-severe AD. The objective of this chapter is to shed light on clinical trials assessing the efficacy of the major novel emerging biologics.

We will focus on dupilumab, an anti-IL4 and IL13 antibody, tralokinumab, an anti-IL-13 antibody, lebrikizumab that binds specifically to soluble IL-13, neomizumab, an anti-IL-31 antibody, eblazakimab, an IL-13R-alpha-1 monoclonal antibody, and agents targeting OX40/OX40L.

2. Biologics

A summary of biologics is presented in **Table 1**.

2.1 Dupilumab

Despite the presence of a multitude of newly emerging drugs, the approval of dupilumab, is the major breakthrough in managing moderate to severe AD in the last decade. Dupilumab has been evaluated in many randomized clinical trials, prospective cohort studies, and meta-analyses.

2.1.1 Meta-analysis

A network meta-analysis [2] demonstrated with a high degree of certainty that dupilumab is the most effective treatment in achieving EASI-75 (risk ratio 3.04, 95% CI 2.51–3.69) and improving the POEM score (mean difference 7.3, 95% CI 6.61–8.00) during short-term follow-up when compared with placebo. This meta-analysis was performed on 74 randomized trials with >8000 participants. Moreover, in achieving EASI-75 and the score of POEM, dupilumab ranked first compared to other investigational and noninvestigational biologics. However, due to a lack of head-to-head studies, ranking of nonivestigational drugs with respect to dupilumab is not possible.

2.1.2 SOLO1 and SOLO2 studies

SOLO1 (671 patients) and SOLO2 (708 patients) are two identically-designed randomized, placebo-controlled, phase 3 trials in adults with moderate-to-severe atopic dermatitis, inadequately controlled by topical treatment [3]. Patients were randomly assigned for 16 weeks to receives: either 300 mg dupilumab weekly or placebo weekly or 300 mg of dupilumab every other week alternating with placebo. The primary outcome of the studies was the proportion of patients with a score of 0 (clear) or 1 (almost clear) on the Investigator's Global Assessment (IGA) and a reduction of 2 points or more in IGA from baseline at the end of the study.

Drug	Mode of action	Current phase of clinical trial and approvals	Dose and frequency	Baseline laboratory workup	Follow-up workup	Side effects	Contraindications or precautions
Monoclonal antibodies							
Dupilumab	Fully human monoclonal antibody that binds to the alpha subunit of the IL-4 receptor and inhibits downstream signaling of IL-4 and IL-13	FDA approved for moderate-to-severe AD in: • adults and children ≥12 y.o (2017) • children 6–12 y.o (2021) • children 6 months-6 y.o (2022) • FDA approved for patients ≥6 months old	≥18 y.o: initial loading dose: 600 mg SC injection followed by 300 mg Q2W. 6–18[y.o: ≥60 kg: 600 mg loading dose then 300 mg Q2W 30–60[kg: 400 mg loading dose then 200 mg Q2W 15–30[kg: 600 mg loading dose then 300 mg Q4W 6 months-6[y.o: 15–30[kg NO loading. 300 mg Q4W 5–15[kg: NO loading. 200 mg Q4W	None	None	• injection site reaction • ocular surface disease (11–26%): conjunctivitis and, infrequently, keratitis, eye dryness, burning or stinging, pruritus, blepharitis, and blurred vision • Seronegative arthritis and enthesitis/enthesopathy: psoriasis and inflammatory arthritis and enthesitis, associated, paradoxical emergence of T helper type 17 (Th17) diseases (spondyloarthropathy-pattern arthritis, psoriasiform skin disease, and occasional anterior uveitis.) • Exacerbation or new onset of head and neck dermatitis (4–10%) • antibody development against the drug • eosinophilia • herpes simplex virus infection (ex: oral herpes) • upper respiratory tract, skin infection	• Pregnancy: limited data. Risk-benefit balance • Lactation: limited data. Risk-benefit balance • renal insufficiency: no adjustment for mild-to-moderate renal impairment. No data if severe. • hepatic insufficiency: no data • Parasitic (helminth infections): Patients with known helminth infections were excluded from clinical studies. It is unknown if dupilumab might influence immune response against helminth infections. Treat patients with pre-existing helminth infections before initiating dupilumab. If patients become infected while on dupilumab and do not respond to antihelminth treatment, discontinue dupilumab until infection resolves. • Vaccinations: Consider completing all age-appropriate vaccinations. Avoid live vaccines. Unknown if efficacy or safety of vaccine will be altered with dupilumab

Drug	Mode of action	Current phase of clinical trial and approvals	Dose and frequency	Baseline laboratory workup	Follow-up workup	Side effects	Contraindications or precautions
Tralokinumab	Fully human monoclonal anti-IL-13 antibody	FDA approved for moderate-to-severe AD in: Adults ≥18 y.o (2021)	initial loading dose: 600 mg SC injection followed by 300 mg Q2W, or Q4W may be considered in patients <100 kg who achieve clear or almost clear skin after 16 weeks of treatment	None	None	• viral upper respiratory tract infection (15%) • ocular surface disease (5.6%) • injection-site reactions (3/5%) • eosinophilia • atopic dermatitis exacerbation	Same as dupilumab
Lebrikizumab	Monoclonal antibody that binds specifically to soluble IL-13	Not yet FDA approved	initial loading dose: 500 mg SC injection followed by 250 mg Q2W			• atopic dermatitis exacerbation (9%) • ocular surface disease (8%) nasopharyngitis (8%) • Herpes infection • eosinophilia	
Nemolizumab	Humanized monoclonal antibody against the receptor of IL-31, a cytokine known to be associated with pruritus via IL-31 receptor activation	Not yet FDA approved	Yet to be determined.			• atopic dermatitis exacerbation • respiratory tract infections • peripheral edema • elevated CPK • injection site reactions • headache • GI symptoms	

Table 1.
Summary of biologics in atopic dermatitis.

In SOLO 1, the primary outcome occurred in 85 patients (38%) on dupilumab every 2 weeks, in 83 on dupilumab weekly (37%), vs. 10% (n = 23) on placebo ($p < 0.001$ for each vs. placebo).

In SOLO 2, the primary outcome occurred in 84 patients (36%) on dupilumab every other week, in 36% (n = 87) receiving dupilumab weekly, vs. 8% (n = 20) receiving placebo ($p < 0.001$ for both comparisons).

In SOLO1 and SOLO2, EASI-75 was achieved in significantly more patients receiving each regimen of dupilumab than in those receiving placebo ($p < 0.001$ for all comparisons). In addition, dupilumab was also associated with a reduction in itch, anxiety or depression, and improvement in quality of life.

2.1.3 LIBERTY AD CHRONOS study

LIBERTY AD CHRONOS is a randomized, double-blind, trial that aimed to study long-term efficacy and safety of dupilumab [4]. Patients were randomly assigned to receive dupilumab 300 mg once weekly or dupilumab 300 mg every 2 weeks or placebo for 52 weeks. A concurrent treatment with topical steroids was given to all patients. The two coprimary endpoints were the proportion of patients with both an IGA score of 0 or 1 or at least 2 point reduction and the proportion of patients achieving EASI-75 at the end of the study. At the end, more patients in the dupilumab groups achieved both: the IGA endpoint and EASI-75 vs. placebo (40 versus 13%, and 65 versus 22%, respectively).

2.1.4 Other studies

An open-label, extension study [5] examined 1491 patients enrolled in previous studies given 300 mg of dupilumab every week for up to 76 weeks at data cutoff. While the primary outcome was safety, efficacy was also evaluated. Among 1491 enrolled, 92.9% were receiving treatment at cutoff. The safety profile was consistent with previously reported trials, with no new safety signals. Among the common adverse events, we note: nasopharyngitis, conjunctivitis, and cutaneous reactions at the site of injection. Sustained improvement was seen up to 76 weeks, with >60% achieving EASI-90 scores at 56 and 76 weeks.

2.2 Tralokinumab

2.2.1 ECZTRA 1 and ECZTRA 2 studies

ECZTRA 1 and ECZTRA 2 are 2 identical randomized trials, in which 1596 adult patients with moderate-to-severe AD were randomized to receive either subcutaneous tralokinumab 300 mg every 2 weeks or placebo [6]. Primary endpoints were a score of 0 or 1 in IGA and EASI 75 at the 16th week. Patients achieving an IGA score of 0 or 1 and/or EASI 75 with tralokinumab at the end of the 16th week were rerandomized to receive either tralokinumab Q2W or tralokinumab every 4 weeks or placebo, for another 36 weeks. An IGA score of 0/1 was achieved by 16% in tralokinumab vs. 7% placebo in ECZTRA 1 and 22% in tralokinumab vs. 11% in placebo in ECZTRA 2. EASI-75 was achieved by 25 vs. 13% and 33 vs. 11% in these 2 studies, respectively. Tralokinumab was also more effective than placebo in reducing the SCORAD score, improving pruritus, and improving quality of life. The majority of tralokinumab responders at week 16 maintained response at week 52 with continued treatment.

2.2.2 ECZTRA 3 study

ECZTRA 3 is a trial in which 380 patients were assigned to receive either tralokinumab 300 mg every 2 weeks or placebo in combination with a topical corticosteroid applied as needed [7]. At 16 weeks, the IGA score 0/1 was 39 vs. 26% and EASI-75 was 56 vs. 36% for tralokinumab vs. placebo, respectively. Similar results were observed with concomitant topical corticosteroid use in adults previously treated with cyclosporine (ECZTRA 7 study).

In a meta-analysis of >16,000 participants (60 clinical trials), tralokinumab was found to be slightly less effective than dupilumab in reducing EASI at the same dose at week 16 [8].

2.3 Lebrikizumab

2.3.1 ADhere study

ADhere study is a 16-week randomized, double-blinded, placebo-controlled, and multicentre study on moderate-to-severe AD patients [9]. 211 adults and adolescents were assigned to receive lebrikizumab (loading dose of 500 mg at baseline and week 2, followed by 250 mg every 2 weeks) in combination with low- to mid-potency topical corticosteroids vs. placebo. The proportion of those in the drug group achieving an IGA score of 0/1 at week 16 was higher (41% vs. 22%).

2.3.2 ADvocate1 and ADvocate2 studies

ADvocate1 and ADvocate2 are identical trials in which 851 adults and adolescents with moderate-to-severe AD were assigned to receive either lebrikizumab (loading dose of 500 mg at baseline followed by 250 mg every other week) or placebo [10]. More patients in the lebrikizumab groups achieved an IGA score of 0/1 at week 16 (43 vs. 13% and 33 vs. 11%).

In an extension study of the ADvocate1 and ADvocate2 studies, 71% in the group lebrikizumab every 2 weeks, 77% in the group lebrikizumab every 4 weeks, and 48% in the placebo group achieved an IGA score of 0/1 at week 52 [11].

2.4 Nemolizumab

- A phase 2, randomized, double-blind, and 12-week study [12] was conducted assigning patients to receive either nemolizumab (0.1, 0.5 mg, or 2 mg/kg) or placebo every 4 weeks or nemolizumab 2 mg/kg every 8 weeks. The primary end point was the improvement in the score on the pruritus visual-analogue. Secondary end points were EASI and BSA of AD. Pruritus was reduced by 44%, 60%, and 63% in the nemolizumab 0.1, 0.5, and 2 mg groups, respectively, compared to the placebo group with 21%. The BSA of AD decreased by 8, 20, and 19% in nemolizumab groups, vs. 16% in the placebo group.

- A Japanese randomized trial [13] including 215 patients ≥13 y.o with AD and moderate to severe pruritus were assigned to receive either nemolizumab 60 mg or placebo every 4 weeks for 16 weeks plus topical therapy. At week 16, the least squares mean of the pruritus visual analogue scale score was reduced by 43% in the treated group vs. 21% in the placebo.

Although studies are promising regarding the use of neomizumab in moderate-to-severe atopic dermatitis, more studies are needed to evaluate its safety and long-term efficacy.

2.5 Eblasakimab

Eblasakimab is an IL-13R-alpha-1 monoclonal antibody currently being evaluated in a phase 2b randomized clinical trial. Early data presented at the American Academy of Dermatology 2022 showed significant efficacy after 8 weeks of treatment in a small sample size of patients that were assigned to receive eblasakimab 200 mg, 400 mg, or 600 mg vs. placebo. A significant EASI reduction was noted: 61% with 600 mg, 63% with 400 mg group, and 50% with 200 mg. EASI 50 was achieved in 77%, 71%, and 50% of patients in the respective eblasakimab groups vs. 38% in the placebo group. EASI 75 was achieved in 50%, 57%, and 50% with eblasakimab groups, vs. 13% in the placebo group. Moreover, the peak pruritus NRS decreased by 37% with eblasakimab 600 mg, vs. 16% with placebo [14].

2.6 Agents targeting OX40/OX40L

Agents binding to OX40, a costimulatory receptor on activated T cells (telazorlimab and rocatinlimab) or to the OX40 ligand (amlitelimab) have been evaluated in phase 2 studies in adults. Rocatinlimab, was evaluated in a study phase 2b that was placebo-controlled. At week 16, groups receiving rocatinlimab achieved a reduction in the EASI greater than the placebo (−48.3% to −61.1%). There was a sustained response up to 20 weeks after the treatment was stopped. Amlitelimab was studied in a phase 2a clinical trial, at week 16, amlitelimab groups reached the EASI mean percentage – 69.9% and – 80.1% versus the placebo (−49.4%). Both treatments were shown to be safe and well tolerated [15, 16]

3. Conclusion

New biologics have been developed in the treatment of moderate-to-severe AD and have displayed outstanding efficacy [17].

Recent studies have elucidated the mechanism of AD by characterizing various phenotypes and endotypes. Emerging topical and systemic narrow-targeting treatments have been developed according to these findings.

Emerging topical and systemic targeted agents, which have displayed safety and efficacy, are being developed on the basis of expanding knowledge of the pathophysiology of this disease. On the other hand, upcoming clinical trials will provide data for additional options in AD treatments. These new therapies might raise problems like long-term socioeconomic burden associated with biologics. We are currently at the dawn of a new era in the treatment of AD.

Author details

Charbel Skayem[1,2*] and Tu Anh Duong[3,4,5]

1 Faculty of Medicine, Sorbonne University, Paris, France

2 Paris Saclay University, Hôpitaux de Paris (AP-HP), Paris, France

3 Telemedicine Department, Paris Saclay University, Assistance Publique Hôpitaux de Paris (AP-HP), Paris, France

4 Chaire Avenir Santé numérique, Paris, France

5 Research Group Dynamyc, Paris, France

*Address all correspondence to: charbelskayem@hotmail.com

References

[1] Yamamura K, Nakahara T. The Dawn of a new era in atopic dermatitis treatment. Journal of Clinical Medicine. 2022;**11**(20):6145. DOI: 10.3390/jcm11206145

[2] Sawangjit R, Dilokthornsakul P, Lloyd-Lavery A, et al. Systemic treatments for eczema: A network meta-analysis. Cochrane Database of Systematic Reviews. 2020;**9**:CD013206

[3] Simpson EL, Bieber T, Guttman-Yassky E, et al. Two phase 3 trials of Dupilumab versus placebo in atopic dermatitis. The New England Journal of Medicine. 2016;**375**:2335

[4] Blauvelt A, de Bruin-Weller M, Gooderham M, et al. Long-term management of moderate-to-severe atopic dermatitis with dupilumab and concomitant topical corticosteroids (LIBERTY AD CHRONOS): A 1-year, randomised, double-blinded, placebo-controlled, phase 3 trial. Lancet. 2017;**389**:2287

[5] Deleuran M, Thaçi D, Beck LA, de Bruin-Weller M, Blauvelt A, Forman S, et al. Dupilumab shows long-term safety and efficacy in patients with moderate to severe atopic dermatitis enrolled in a phase 3 open-label extension study. Journal of the American Academy of Dermatology. 2020;**82**(2):377-388. DOI: 10.1016/j.jaad.2019.07.074

[6] Wollenberg A, Blauvelt A, Guttman-Yassky E, Worm M, Lynde C, Lacour JP, et al. ECZTRA 1 and ECZTRA 2 study investigators. Tralokinumab for moderate-to-severe atopic dermatitis: results from two 52-week, randomized, double-blind, multicentre, placebo-controlled phase III trials (ECZTRA 1 and ECZTRA 2). British Journal of Dermatology. 2021;**184**(3):437-449. DOI: 10.1111/bjd.19574

[7] Silverberg JI, Toth D, Bieber T, Alexis AF, Elewski BE, Pink AE, et al. ECZTRA 3 study investigators. Tralokinumab plus topical corticosteroids for the treatment of moderate-to-severe atopic dermatitis: Results from the double-blind, randomized, multicentre, placebo-controlled phase III ECZTRA 3 trial. The British Journal of Dermatology. 2021;**184**(3):450-463. DOI: 10.1111/bjd.19573

[8] Drucker AM, Morra DE, Prieto-Merino D, Ellis AG, Yiu ZZN, Rochwerg B, et al. Systemic immunomodulatory treatments for atopic dermatitis: Update of a living systematic review and network Meta-analysis. JAMA Dermatology. 2022;**158**(5):523-532. DOI: 10.1001/jamadermatol.2022.0455

[9] Simpson EL, Gooderham M, Wollenberg A, Weidinger S, Armstrong A, Soung J, et al. Efficacy and safety of lebrikizumab in combination with topical corticosteroids in adolescents and adults with moderate-to-severe atopic dermatitis: A Randomized Clinical Trial (ADhere). JAMA Dermatology. 2023;**159**(2):182-191. DOI: 10.1001/jamadermatol.2022.5534 Erratum in: JAMA Dermatol. 2023 Sep 1;159(9):1014

[10] Silverberg JI, Guttman-Yassky E, Thaçi D, Irvine AD, Stein Gold L, Blauvelt A, et al. ADvocate1 and ADvocate2 investigators. Two phase 3 trials of Lebrikizumab for moderate-to-severe atopic dermatitis. The New England Journal of Medicine. 2023;**388**(12):1080-1091. DOI: 10.1056/NEJMoa2206714

[11] Blauvelt A, Thyssen JP, Guttman-Yassky E, Bieber T, Serra-Baldrich E, Simpson E, et al. Efficacy and safety of lebrikizumab in moderate-to-severe atopic dermatitis: 52-week results of two randomized double-blinded placebo-controlled phase III trials. The British Journal of Dermatology. 2023;**188**(6): 740-748. DOI: 10.1093/bjd/ljad022

[12] Ruzicka T, Hanifin JM, Furue M, Pulka G, Mlynarczyk I, Wollenberg A, et al. Anti-Interleukin-31 receptor A antibody for atopic dermatitis. The New England Journal of Medicine. 2017;**376**(9):826-835. DOI: 10.1056/NEJMoa1606490

[13] Kabashima K, Matsumura T, Komazaki H, Kawashima M, Nemolizumab-JP01 Study Group. Trial of Nemolizumab and topical agents for atopic dermatitis with pruritus. The New England Journal of Medicine. 2020;**383**(2):141-150. DOI: 10.1056/NEJMoa1917006

[14] Blauvelt A. *Eblasakimab*, a human anti-IL-13 receptor monoclonal antibody, in adult patients with moderate-to-severe atopic dermatitis: A randomized, double-blinded, placebo-controlled, proof-of-concept study. In: Proceedings of the American Academy of Dermatology Annual Meeting; Boston, MA, USA, 26 March 2022

[15] Guttman-Yassky E, Esfandiari E, Chong C, Matsui T, Mano H. Rocatinlimab* (AMG 451/KHK4083) demonstrates improvements in head and neck atopic dermatitis in patients with moderate-severe disease in A Phase 2 Trial. In: Proceedings of the 31st European Academy of Dermatology and Venereology (EADV) Congress, Virtual Meeting; Milan, Italy, 7-10 September 2022

[16] Weidinger S, Cork M, Reich A, Bieber T, Gilber S, Brennan N, et al. Treatment with Amlitelimab – A novel non-depleting, non-cytotoxic antiOX40Ligand monoclonal antibody–reduces IL-22 serum levels in a Phase 2a Randomized, Placebo-Controlled Trial in patients with moderate-to-severe atopic dermatitis. In: Proceedings of the 31st European Academy of Dermatology and Venereology (EADV) Congress 2022; Milan, Italy, 7-10 September 2022

[17] Howe W, Paller A, Butala S. Treatment of atopix dermatitis (eczema). Uptodate. 2023

Chapter 5

New Treatments and Validations for Atopic Dermatitis in Humans after Comparative Approach with Canine Models

Rosanna Marsella

Abstract

This chapter aims to open doors to novel treatments of human Atopic Dermatitis (AD) after validation of successful response in canine AD. Dogs are currently the best model for the human disease and research in this species can benefit people. Interestingly, treatment options used in dogs (e.g., Allergen-specific immunotherapy, oral Janus Kinase Inhibitor and of a biologic targeting Interleukin-31) have equivalents in human medicine. Areas of interest for the future should focus on increasing the efficacy of allergen-specific immunotherapy, modulating non-specific immune response, restoring of cutaneous and gut microbiome by topical application or fecal transplant, and using stem cell therapy. The overall goal is to find treatments that are safe and sustainable to avoid broad spectrum immunosuppressive medications and repair bacterial imbalances in order to minimize the use of antibiotics in these patients.

Keywords: atopic dermatitis, dogs, humans, JAK inhibitors, IL-31, biologics, stem cell, microbiome

1. Introduction

Canine atopic dermatitis (AD) has many similarities with the human counterpart both clinically and immunologically. For this reason, canine AD has been considered the best current model for the human disease [1] and many treatments used to treat canine patients are either used in human medicine or have great potential to be considered for people [2]. Dogs, like people, develop a chronic pruritic inflammatory disease that affects specific areas of the body and are prone to Staphylococcal infections which further aggravate the severity of pruritus. The disease in dogs is chronic progressive and it is associated in most cases with allergic sensitization to either foods or environmental allergens. The main route of sensitization in dogs is epicutaneous as the skin barrier function in atopic dogs is altered [3], similar to what is the case in people [4, 5]. Skin barrier defects have been documented in atopic dogs [6] and play an important role in disease development, as they do in humans [7, 8]. Since inflammation worsens skin barrier, these changes are progressive and promote additional sensitization in the lifetime of the patient [9]. Canine atopic patients undergo frequent course of antibiotics and are frequently affected by resistant infections. Thus, control of the disease is critical for both the quality of life of the animal and the owners, as well as to minimize the development and transmission of multidrug resistant bacteria.

As it is in people, the canine disease is multifactorial and the result of a combination of genetic and environmental factors. Atopic dermatitis in dogs has become increasingly common in westernized countries in the last few decades either because of increased awareness or because of changed life-style conditions. Processed foods, excessive exposure to indoor environments with dust mites, and decreased exposure to outdoor farm environments have been considered risk factors in dogs [10] as they are considered for people [11].

Similarly to humans, atopic dogs have less biodiversity in their cutaneous [12, 13] and gut microbiome [14, 15]. Skin microbiome dysbiosis in atopic dogs is particularly exacerbated during allergen induced flares [16]. Dysbiosis is also a hallmark of human AD [17] leading to a prominent Th2 response and a decreased regulatory response [18]. Significant efforts have been devoted to increase biodiversity and normalize the immune response, by either application of beneficial bacteria on the skin [19] or by fecal transplant [20, 21]. The latter has recently been tried in clinical patients in human medicine with encouraging results [22]. Since all these factors (diet, microbiome, skin barrier, sensitization to environmental allergens) are all interconnected, the approach to address canine AD has been multimodal and has relied on a variety of strategies ranging from symptomatic control of the inflammation, to skin barrier repair strategies, and allergen specific immunotherapy to address sensitization developed by the patient and promote tolerance.

Interestingly some treatments have been available first in veterinary medicine (e.g., oral Janus Kinase inhibitor for AD and biologic targeting IL-31) before an equivalent was approved in human medicine while for other medications, the opposite has been true. The advantage of testing treatment in dogs is that approval of studies is, on average, faster and easier and useful information can be obtained that can benefit both canine and human patients. As many atopic humans are children, testing of new strategies in dogs first is an appealing approach.

1.1 Currently approved treatments for canine AD

The clinical approach to canine AD includes short-term strategies to decrease pruritus and inflammation as well as long-term strategies to decrease the need of rescue medications and the severity of flares. Under the short-term strategies are the medications that rapidly and primarily address allergic cytokines. In this category, the most commonly used are glucocorticoids (either topically or systemically) and oclacitinib, a Janus Kinase (JAK) inhibitor.

Oclacitinib is an oral selective JAK1 inhibitor that targets the signaling of cytokines important for allergic inflammation [23]. The selectivity for JAK1 and the blockage of signaling of cytokines that are important for allergic inflammation rather than for innate immunity and hematopoiesis, are important considerations for the safety profile of oclacitinib. These characteristics make oclacitinib different from many of the initially approved JAK inhibitors in human medicine, drugs that target other JAK/STAT signaling pathways [24].

The speed of action of glucocorticoids and oclacitinib is comparable and measurable within a few hours after administration [25] thus, both strategies are suitable to quick relief from pruritus. Oclacitinib has been shown to significantly improve the quality of life of allergic dogs [26] and is not associated with increased risk of cancer [27]. This is an important difference between the use of JAK inhibitors in human medicine and oclacitinib in veterinary medicine. Many systemic JAK inhibitors in people have been used for the treatment of rheumatoid arthritis, inflammatory bowel disease, transplant rejection, and psoriasis [28]. In humans with rheumatoid arthritis and other autoimmune diseases, independent of the type of treatment, there is a concern for increased risk of certain malignancies [29, 30].

The JAK inhibitors currently considered for AD in people are topicals (e.g., ruxolitinib cream and delgocitinib ointment). Oral options (e.g., baricitinib (JAK1/2), abrocitinib (JAK1-selective), and upadacitinib (JAK1-selective) have been associated with nausea, headache, upper respiratory tract infection, and to a lesser degree, herpes infections [31]. No topical JAK inhibitor is currently available in veterinary medicine.

Another approach to canine AD and pruritus is the use of an injectable biologic, lokivetmab, that specifically targets canine Interleukin 31 (IL-31). IL-31 is a cytokine that has received a lot of interest in recent years for its role in mediating pruritus and allergic inflammation [32, 33]. Lokivetmab is a caninized monoclonal antibody that targets canine IL-31. Lokivetmab takes a few hours to days to work and may not work in all patients, but it is commonly used in clinical practice as either a monotherapy or an adjunctive therapy. In some patients that benefit may be seen in a few hours and duration seems to be dose dependent [34, 35]. Lokivetmab has also shown usefulness as a tool for a proactive control of the disease [36]. A proactive approach is becoming more popular in both veterinary and human medicine since atopic patients are prone to relapses. Treating the disease once the relapse has occurred requires more medications and drugs of a broader spectrum of action to induce remission. Instead, a proactive long-term maintenance regimen leads to increased time to flare and decreased need for rescue medications [37, 38]. In that context, lokivetmab is adopted more and more frequently by veterinarians to keep patients comfortable.

In human medicine, there is currently no approved monoclonal targeting IL-31 but there is an anti-IL-31 receptor α-chain (IL-31RA) monoclonal antibody, nemolizumab [39]. Interestingly, trials for biologics targeting human IL-31 have been registered, but no results have been published at this time; thus, the caninized monoclonal against IL-31 does not have an equivalent in human medicine.

Among treatments that require longer time to work and control canine AD are drugs such as cyclosporine, which may take 3–4 weeks to start working [40]. Cyclosporine is used for long-term symptomatic control of allergic dogs [41] and, prior to the development of oclacitinib and lokivetmab, was one of the most commonly prescribed treatments. Many dogs develop severe gastrointestinal adverse effects [42] and chronic use increases the risk of saprophytic infections [43, 44]. Cyclosporine is also used for severe cases of AD in people although some of the new biologics are decreasing its use [45, 46].

For the long-term control of canine AD, Allergen Specific Immunotherapy (ASIT) is frequently recommended [47]. It requires several months and is considered a long-term approach to reeducate the immune system and halt the progression of the disease. Allergen specific immunotherapy is used for patients with a long season and can be administered by various routes ranging from injectable to sublingual and intralymphatic, depending on formulations of allergens available in the specific country and the preferences of the owners and the clinician. In dogs, in the US, the most commonly used route of administration of the allergen has been subcutaneous while in Europe intralymphatic is done routinely [48, 49]. When the various routes of administration have been compared for efficacy in canine patients, the subcutaneous and the intralymphatic route have shown more efficacy than the sublingual route [50].

Interestingly, ASIT is frequently used for human patients with asthma and rhinitis and venom hypersensitivity [51], but its use for AD in people is not widespread. In fact, ASIT's efficacy in human patients with eczema is still questioned [52]. Only recent studies have shown that ASIT is a beneficial adjunctive therapy for AD patients with allergic sensitizations [53] while in dogs its benefit for AD has been long recognized. In veterinary medicine, the dermatologist is also the allergist; thus, facilitating the process of allergy testing and the formulation of a custom-made vaccine. In human medicine, these are two different figures and AD has been considered for decades more of a disease of skin barrier rather than an allergic disease, thus ASIT is not routinely considered as a long-term strategy to decrease severity of skin flares in atopic patients. It is hoped that this strategy is considered in polysensitized human patients with cutaneous disease.

1.2 Areas of research in canine AD

1.2.1 Strategies to improve immunotherapy

The new treatments have provided new tools to help affected patients, however, there are always some dogs that do not respond or develop adverse effects, thus there are unmet needs and the need to exploration other strategies. Areas of interest include ways to improve the success rate of immunotherapy considering different formulations to increase the desired immune response, or using recombinant allergens to ensure standardization of allergens [54, 55]. Faster response and increased safety are important factors that can enhance compliance with immunotherapy.

Currently, there is minimal standardization of allergen extracts and identification of the most effective protocol in veterinary medicine. As a result, there is a wide range of protocols and doses being used without strong evidence to support one over the other. When efficacy and speed to reach effect with allergen specific immunotherapy in dogs, it was found that efficacy was significantly higher with the polymerized allergoids coupled with non-oxidized mannan than for the "classic" aqueous and alum-precipitated subcutaneous IT types [56]. Allergoids improve safety and formulations using nanoparticles or microparticle packed with the allergen are considered with vehicles that protect immunogenicity to be suitable for oral immunotherapy rather than injectable. Adjuvants that enhance the desired immune response have also been considered [57]. They are typically products derived from Gram-negative bacteria and have been shown to increase Th1 cytokine and regulatory cytokines like IL-10 [58, 59]. Liposome-DNA combined with protein or peptide antigens can be used effectively as a vaccine adjuvant and in pilot studies liposome-DNA complexes mixed with allergen had beneficial effect on pruritus [60].

In dogs, several studies have been published using cytosine-phosphate-guanine oligodeoxynucleotides bound to gelatine nanoparticles as immunotherapy for canine AD [61, 62] as strategy to induce gamma Interferon (IFN-γ) and improve clinical efficacy. Cytosine-phosphate-guanine oligodeoxynucleotides (CpG ODN) are short single-stranded synthetic DNA molecules that bind to the Toll-like receptor 9 on antigen presenting cells and promote the release of IFN-γ, TNF, IL-6, and IL-12 and suppress Th2 response.

The question whether immunotherapy needs to be allergen specific is an important one as non-allergen specific strategies could be of great benefit. This approach would typically include inactivated bacterial products aimed to increase a regulatory response. This approach is considered palatable to help patients where owners do not have the resources to do allergy testing which is necessary for a custom made "vaccine". Injection of killed bacterial products has shown promise in veterinary medicine. In one double-blinded, placebo-controlled study, 64 atopic dogs were allocated to receive intradermal injection of a suspension of heat-killed mycobacterium vaccae or placebo [63]. Dogs with mild to moderate disease showed improvement while it did not help, as monotherapy, more severe cases. Interestingly, when the same strategy was used in children with AD no benefit could be found [64, 65]. Another killed bacterial formulation used in veterinary medicine has been a suspension of *Gordonia bronchialis*, *Rhodococcus coprophilus*, or *Tsukamurella inchonensis*. Injection of two doses, three weeks apart from each other of this mix of Actinomycetales has been effective in decreasing severity of lesions and pruritus in dogs allergic to fleas [66]. This strategy has not been explored yet in human medicine to decrease severity of allergic skin disease.

Bacteriotherapy aims to restore diversity in the microbiome of atopic patients and is being explored to decrease severity of allergic skin disease and decrease the need for chronic antibiotic therapy. Skin bacterial transplants have been attempted and results have been encouraging in people [67]. Topical application of benign staphylococcus for example has been shown to displace more pathogenic staphylococcus (e.g., *S. aureus*) [68]. No similar study has been published in veterinary medicine.

1.2.2 Anti-pruritics that do not target allergic inflammation

New strategies include exploration of medications that target itch in a broader sense rather than simply focusing on allergic inflammation [69, 70]. Under this category, current studies have considered agonists of cannabinoid receptors as a strategy to decrease pruritus. Dogs, like people, have receptor for cannabinoids [71] in the skin and agonists of those receptors have shown promise in decreasing pruritus. For example, in a prospective, randomized, controlled study, a topical endocannabinoid membrane transporter inhibitor (WOL067–531) minimized allergic flares and pruritus in a canine model of AD [72]. In prospective randomized double-blinded controlled study, using privately owned dogs diagnosed with AD, a mix CBD/CBDA was given orally at 2 mg/kg dose and showed a beneficial effect on pruritus but not on skin lesions [73]. There are also reports of case series of canine patients who were treated with CBD-derived products in conjunction with other therapies that shown beneficial effects. In veterinary medicine, there are several reports on this type of approach to decrease allergic pruritus as adjunctive therapy [74]. Interestingly, few studies have considered this approach for human AD although preliminary reports are encouraging in people as well [75]. Beneficial effects of inflammatory skin diseases have been reported but no controlled studies have been published [76–78].

Similarly, an agonist of K-opioid receptor, asimadoline, has shown promises in a canine study [79] and just recently a synthetic peptide agonist of the kappa opioid receptor has been approved [80]. This medication is for intravenous use, whereas the agonist studied in the canine study was a topical product.

The need to consider different mechanisms and receptors comes from the fact that some pruritic allergic dogs are refractory to commonly used medications. This lack of response may be due to the fact that AD is a clinical syndrome rather than a single disease, and different patients may have different responses to medications, particularly when the mechanism of action is targeted and not broad spectrum.

1.2.3 Modulation of cytokines and administration of recombinant cytokines

The use of biologics to block either a cytokine or a receptor is appealing due to the targeted nature. However, cytokines are pleiotropic, meaning that they can have multiple effects on different processes simultaneously, and they are also redundant, which means that blocking one cytokine may not be sufficient as other cytokines can compensate for the block. As the production of biologics can be challenging and expensive, an alternative approach considered is the actual administration of cytokines to modulate the immune response. Interest in the use of interferons has been expressed in both veterinary and human medicine [81, 82].

In veterinary medicine, most studies have a small number of patients and have used recombinant IFN-γ injectable compared to antihistamine as a positive control and demonstrated more pronounced beneficial effect with the IFN-γ [83]. The effect was found to be dose dependent with the 5000 U/Kg being more effective than 2000 U/kg and several dogs in the higher dose group being in remission for a year after the end of the study [84]. Interferon-omega (IFN-ω) has also been evaluated and its efficacy was found to be comparable to the one of cyclosporine over the course of 6 months in a randomized controlled trial [85]. To overcome the issue of injections, oral administration of IFN has also been considered and compared to injectable when using IFN-ω of a different species (e.g., Feline IFN) [86]. The authors found that both routes of administration led to clinical improvement but significant difference between baseline and end of the study was only achieved in the group that received oral IFN. This consideration is important as oral administration of cytokines although probably degraded in the stomach can still lead to beneficial immune modulation and could increase compliance and access to treatment. No equivalent study has been published in human medicine.

Recombinant human IFN-alfa (IFN-α) was also tested in dogs with AD and the oral route was compared to the subcutaneous route [87]. Although the study was very small, the dogs given IFN orally showed some improvement while injection of IFN was poorly tolerated and needed to be discontinued due to fever, vomiting, and diarrhea.

1.2.4 Stem cells

Mesenchymal stem cells have been considered in both human [88, 89] and veterinary medicine [90] as a promising new treatment of AD due to their immunoregulatory properties. Mesenchymal stem cells are pluripotent, undifferentiated stem cells found in adult tissues have strong anti-inflammatory and immunomodulatory effects on both B and T cells [91, 92]. In an initial small, non-controlled, pilot study, intravenously administered autogenous adipose-derived stem cells (1.3 million cells/kg, one dose) did not significantly decrease pruritus and severity of dermatitis in atopic dogs [93]. Another group reported that intravenous administration of the allogenic canine adipose-derived mesenchymal stem cells (1.5 million cells/kg bodyweight, one dose) to 26 dogs with refractory AD resulted in the remission of clinical signs [94]. Twenty-two animals completed the study. Pruritus and dermatitis scores decreased significantly after one week or month of treatment, respectively, and remained stable for six months. No adverse effects were reported. Multiple intravenous administrations (2 million cells/kg, every 21 days for 3 times) showed beneficial effects in severity of pruritus and dermatitis [95]. All these initial studies lacked a placebo control group.

A more recent study was a double-blinded, placebo-controlled study on the efficacy of adipose-derived allogenic canine mesenchymal stem cells [96] for canine AD. In that study a normal dog was used as a donor and stem cells were injected at 30-day interval for 3 times in multiple body locations in atopic dogs. Severity of disease was monitored for 180 days. The authors reported that the treatment decreased the degree of pruritus and associated signs but that repeated injections may be needed on a monthly basis to maintain clinical benefits. Intramuscular route was investigated as well. In one study, multidose intramuscular allogeneic adipose stem cells (0.5 million per dose) decreased severity of disease and no adverse reactions were observed at the site of injection [97].

Currently, in the USA, there are no stem cell products approved in people as the belief is that stem cells require the destruction of a life. Most of the studies in veterinary medicine have used stem cells derived by adipose tissue either from the same patient or a healthy donor. Yet, the approval of stem cell products is a challenge, thus interest is shifting toward alternative options with similar properties. To overcome the issue of administration of cells, the concept of exosomes has drawn attention. Exosomes are nano-sized vesicles that can travel between cells and deliver their contents. These extracellular vesicles represent an alternative mechanism used by mesenchymal stem cells with strong anti-inflammatory properties [98]. This approach has been tried in mouse models and has resulted in clinical improvement of signs of AD [99]. No studies have been published using atopic dogs.

2. Conclusions

Much progress has been made in the treatment of AD in the past few years, both in human and veterinary medicine. Despite the development of new therapies, there is still the need to identify more options since some patients are unresponsive to currently available choices. Additionally, we need treatments that do not simply mask the clinical signs but that can safely reshape the immune response. In that context, allergen specific immunotherapy is the prime example of a strategy that could be utilized more frequently in human medicine. Although this approach requires months and is not a quick fix, it can halt the progression of the disease and decrease the sensitizations that a patient develops over the course of a life time. While this concept is well accepted for respiratory disease in people, the recommendation of allergen specific immunotherapy for skin disease is underutilized. Based on the experience in veterinary medicine, this approach is very beneficial.

JAK inhibitors that are JAK1selective are another appealing option, either topically or systemically. The experience in veterinary medicine with oclacitinib has been very encouraging and shows that this category of medication can provide great improvement in the quality of life of patients.

Exploration of anti-pruritic that targets non-allergic pruritus is also needed. Studies in human medicine on CBD-derived products is encouraging and it is believed that controlled prospective studies are also done in human medicine to provide more science-based recommendations for clinicians. As many products are available now, it is critical to assess and standardize them to provide sound advice to patients.

Lastly, with the current epidemic of inflammatory and autoimmune diseases, future exploration of anti-inflammatory/immunomodulatory broad strategies like the one of exosomes and stem cells is warranted. It may turn-out that our own bodies are the source of the most powerful weapons that we have to counteract allergies and autoimmunity. Standardized exploration of this approach may dramatically change how we treat chronic inflammatory diseases, not just AD. An open-minded approach on the lessons learned in other species is important for progress. As clinicians we treat diseases and the more we learn, the more we realize how similar these conditions are across species and how we can benefit from these parallels.

Conflict of interest

The authors declare no conflict of interest.

Notes/thanks/other declarations

The author would like to thank Dr. Perlstein for reviewing this manuscript.

Author details

Rosanna Marsella
University of Florida, Gainesville, FL, USA

*Address all correspondence to: marsella@ufl.edu

References

[1] Marsella R, Girolomoni G. Canine models of atopic dermatitis: A useful tool with untapped potential. The Journal of Investigative Dermatology. 2009;**129**(10):2351-2357. DOI: 10.1038/jid.2009.98

[2] Santoro D. Therapies in canine atopic dermatitis: An update. The Veterinary Clinics of North America. Small Animal Practice. 2019;**49**(1):9-26. DOI: 10.1016/j.cvsm.2018.08.002

[3] Shimada K, Yoon JS, Yoshihara T, Iwasaki T, Nishifuji K. Increased transepidermal water loss and decreased ceramide content in lesional and non-lesional skin of dogs with atopic dermatitis. Veterinary Dermatology. 2009;**20**(5-6):541-546. DOI: 10.1111/j.1365-3164.2009.00847.x

[4] Montero-Vilchez T, Segura-Fernández-Nogueras MV, Pérez-Rodríguez I, Soler-Gongora M, Martinez-LopezA,Fernández-GonzálezA, et al. Skin barrier function in psoriasis and atopic dermatitis: Transepidermal water loss and temperature as useful tools to assess disease severity. Journal of Clinical Medicine. 2021;**10**(2):359. DOI: 10.3390/jcm10020359

[5] Wärnberg Gerdin S, Lie A, Asarnoj A, Borres MP, Lødrup Carlsen KC, Färdig M, et al. Nordlund BImpaired skin barrier and allergic sensitization in early infancy. Allergy. 2022;**77**(5):1464-1476. DOI: 10.1111/all.15170

[6] Marsella R, Olivry T, Carlotti DN. International Task Force on Canine Atopic Dermatitis Current evidence of skin barrier dysfunction in human and canine atopic dermatitis. Veterinary Dermatology. 2011;**22**(3):239-248. DOI: 10.1111/j.1365-3164.2011.00967.x

[7] Margolis DJ. Atopic dermatitis: Filaggrin and skin barrier dysfunction. The British Journal of Dermatology. 2022;**186**(3):396. DOI: 10.1111/bjd.20946

[8] Drislane C, Irvine AD. The role of filaggrin in atopic dermatitis and allergic disease. Annals of Allergy, Asthma & Immunology. 2020;**124**(1):36-43. DOI: 10.1016/j.anai.2019.10.008

[9] Beck LA, Cork MJ, Amagai M, De Benedetto A, Kabashima K, Hamilton JD, et al. Type 2 inflammation contributes to skin barrier dysfunction in atopic dermatitis. JID Innovations. 2022;**2**(5):100131. DOI: 10.1016/j.xjidi.2022.100131

[10] Harvey ND, Shaw SC, Craigon PJ, Blott SC, England GCW. Environmental risk factors for canine atopic dermatitis: A retrospective large-scale study in Labrador and golden retrievers. Veterinary Dermatology. 2019;**30**(5):396-e119. DOI: 10.1111/vde.12782

[11] Rutkowski K, Sowa P, Rutkowska-Talipska J, Sulkowski S, Rutkowski R. Allergic diseases: The price of civilisational progress. Postepy Dermatological Alergology. 2014;**31**(2):77-83. DOI: 10.5114/pdia.2014.40936

[12] Bradley CW, Morris DO, Rankin SC, Cain CL, Misic AM, Houser T, et al. Longitudinal Evaluation of the Skin Microbiome and Association with Microenvironment and Treatment in Canine Atopic Dermatitis. The Journal of Investigative Dermatology. 2016;**136**(6):1182-1190. DOI: 10.1016/j.jid.2016.01.023

[13] Santoro D, Marsella R, Pucheu-Haston CM, Eisenschenk MN, Nuttall T,

Bizikova P. Review: Pathogenesis of canine atopic dermatitis: Skin barrier and host-micro-organism interaction. Veterinary Dermatology. 2015;**26**(2):84-e25. DOI: 10.1111/vde.12197

[14] Rostaher A, Morsy Y, Favrot C, Unterer S, Schnyder M, Scharl M, et al. Comparison of the gut microbiome between atopic and healthy dogs-preliminary data. Animals (Basel). 2022;**12**(18):2377. DOI: 10.3390/ani12182377

[15] Craig JM. Atopic dermatitis and the intestinal microbiota in humans and dogs. Veterinary Medical Science. 2016;**2**(2):95-105. DOI: 10.1002/vms3.24

[16] Pierezan F, Olivry T, Paps JS, Lawhon SD, Wu J, Steiner JM, et al. The skin microbiome in allergen-induced canine atopic dermatitis. Veterinary Dermatology. 2016;**27**(5):332-e82. DOI: 10.1111/vde.12366

[17] Bjerre RD, Bandier J, Skov L, Engstrand L, Johansen JD. The role of the skin microbiome in atopic dermatitis: A systematic review. The British Journal of Dermatology. 2017;**177**(5):1272-1278. DOI: 10.1111/bjd.15390

[18] Kobayashi T, Imanishi I. Epithelial-immune crosstalk with the skin microbiota in homeostasis and atopic dermatitis - a mini review. Veterinary Dermatology. 2021;**32**(6):533-e147. DOI: 10.1111/vde.13007

[19] Volz T, Skabytska Y, Guenova E, Chen KM, Frick JS, Kirschning CJ, et al. Nonpathogenic bacteria alleviating atopic dermatitis inflammation induce IL-10-producing dendritic cells and regulatory Tr1 cells. The Journal of Investigative Dermatology. 2014;**134**(1):96-104. DOI: 10.1038/jid.2013.291

[20] Alam MJ, Xie L, Yap YA, Marques FZ, Robert R. Manipulating microbiota to treat atopic dermatitis: Functions and therapies. Pathogens. 2022;**11**(6):642. DOI: 10.3390/pathogens11060642

[21] Kim JH, Kim K, Kim W. Gut microbiota restoration through fecal microbiota transplantation: A new atopic dermatitis therapy. Experimental & Molecular Medicine. 2021;**53**(5):907-916. DOI: 10.1038/s12276-021-00627-6

[22] Mashiah J, Karady T, Fliss-Isakov N, Sprecher E, Slodownik D, Artzi O, et al. Clinical efficacy of fecal microbial transplantation treatment in adults with moderate-to-severe atopic dermatitis. Immunity, Inflammation and Disease. 2022;**10**(3):e570. DOI: 10.1002/iid3.570

[23] Gonzales AJ, Bowman JW, Fici GJ, Zhang M, Mann DW, Mitton-Fry M. Oclacitinib (APOQUEL®) is a novel Janus kinase inhibitor with activity against cytokines involved in allergy. Journal of Veterinary Pharmacology and Therapeutics. 2014;**37**(4):317-324. DOI: 10.1111/jvp.12101

[24] Nakashima C, Yanagihara S, Otsuka A. Innovation in the treatment of atopic dermatitis: Emerging topical and oral Janus kinase inhibitors. Allergological International. 2022;**71**(1):40-46. DOI: 10.1016/j.alit.2021.10.004

[25] Gonzales AJ, Fleck TJ, Humphrey WR, Galvan BA, Aleo MM, Mahabir SP, et al. McCall RB.IL-31-induced pruritus in dogs: A novel experimental model to evaluate anti-pruritic effects of canine therapeutics. Veterinary Dermatology. 2016;**27**(1):34-e10. DOI: 10.1111/vde.12280

[26] Cosgrove SB, Cleaver DM, King VL, Gilmer AR, Daniels AE, Wren JA, et al. Long-term compassionate use of oclacitinib in dogs with atopic and allergic skin disease: Safety, efficacy and

quality of life. Veterinary Dermatology. 2015;**26**(3):171-179. DOI: 10.1111/vde.12194

[27] Lancellotti B, Angus J, Edginton H, et al. Age- and breed-matched retrospective co-hort study of malignancies and benign skin masses in 660 dogs with allergic der-matitis treated long-term with versus without oclacitinib. JAVMA. 2020;**257**(5):507-516. DOI: 10.2460/javma.257.5.507

[28] Sivaraman P, Cohen SB. Malignancy and Janus Kinase Inhibition. Rheumatic Diseases Clinics of North America. 2017;**43**:79-93. DOI: 10.1016/j.rdc.2016.09.008

[29] Curtis JR, Lee EB, Kaplan IV, Kwok K, Geier J, Benda B, et al. Tofacitinib, an oral Janus kinase inhibitor: Analysis of malignancies across the rheumatoid arthritis clinical development programme. Annals of the Rheumatic Diseases. 2016;**75**:831-841. DOI: 10.1136/annrheumdis-2014-205,847

[30] Benucci M, Damiani A, Infantino M, Manfredi M, Lari B, Grossi V, et al. Cardiovascular safety, cancer and Jak-inhibitors: Differences to be highlighted. Pharmacological Research. 2022;**183**:106359. DOI: 10.1016/j.phrs.2022.106359

[31] Chovatiya R, Paller AS. JAK inhibitors in the treatment of atopic dermatitis. The Journal of Allergy and Clinical Immunology. 2021;**148**(4):927-940. DOI: 10.1016/j.jaci.2021.08.009

[32] Murdaca G, Greco M, Tonacci A, Negrini S, Borro M, Puppo F, et al. IL-33/IL-31 Axis in Immune-Mediated and Allergic Diseases. International Journal of Molecular Sciences. 2019;**20**(23):5856. DOI: 10.3390/ijms20235856

[33] Datsi A, Steinhoff M, Ahmad F, Alam M, Buddenkotte J. Interleukin-31: The "itchy" cytokine in inflammation and therapy. Allergy. 2021;**76**(10):2982-2997. DOI: 10.1111/all.14791

[34] Souza CP, Rosychuk RAW, Contreras ET, Schissler JR, Simpson AC. A retrospective analysis of the use of lokivetmab in the management of allergic pruritus in a referral population of 135 dogs in the western USA. Veterinary Dermatology. 2018;**29**(6):489-e164. DOI: 10.1111/vde.12682

[35] Fleck TJ, Norris LR, Mahabir S, Walters RR, Martinon O, Dunham SA, et al. Onset and duration of action of lokivetmab in a canine model of IL-31 induced pruritus. Veterinary Dermatology. 2021;**32**(6):681-e182. DOI: 10.1111/vde.12943

[36] Tamamoto-Mochizuki C, Paps JS, Olivry T. Proactive maintenance therapy of canine atopic dermatitis with the anti-IL-31 lokivetmab. Can a monoclonal antibody blocking a single cytokine prevent allergy flares? Veterinary Dermatology. 2019;**30**:98-e26. DOI: 10.1111/vde.12715

[37] Christodoulides P, Hirata Y, Domínguez-Hüttinger E, Danby SG, Cork MJ, Williams HC, et al. Computational design of treatment strategies for proactive therapy on atopic dermatitis using optimal control theory. Philosophical Transactions. Series A, Mathematical, Physical, and Engineering Sciences. 2017;**375**(2096):20160285. DOI: 10.1098/rsta.2016.0285

[38] Lourenço AM, Schmidt V, São Braz B, Nóbrega D, Nunes T, Duarte-Correia JH, et al. Efficacy of proactive long-term maintenance therapy of canine atopic dermatitis with 0.0584% hydrocortisone aceponate spray: A double-blind placebo-controlled pilot study. Veterinary Dermatology. 2016;**27**(2):88-92e25. DOI: 10.1111/vde.12285

[39] Labib A, Vander Does A, Yosipovitch G. Nemolizumab for atopic dermatitis. Drugs Today (Barc). 2022;**58**(4):159-173. DOI: 10.1358/dot.2022.58.4.3378056

[40] Little PR, King VL, Davis KR, Cosgrove SB, Stegemann MR. A blinded, randomized clinical trial comparing the efficacy and safety of oclacitinib and ciclosporin for the control of atopic dermatitis in client-owned dogs. Veterinary Dermatology. 2015;**26**(1):23-30. DOI: 10.1111/vde.12186

[41] Steffan J, Favrot C, Mueller R. A systematic review and meta-analysis of the efficacy and safety of cyclosporin for the treatment of atopic dermatitis in dogs. Veterinary Dermatology. 2000;**17**(1):3-16. DOI: 10.1111/j.1365-3164.2005.00491.x

[42] Archer TM, Boothe DM, Langston VC, Fellman CL, Lunsford KV, Mackin AJ. Oral cyclosporine treatment in dogs: A review of the literature. Journal of Veterinary Internal Medicine. 2014;**28**(1):1-20. DOI: 10.1111/jvim.12265

[43] Radowicz SN. Long-term use of cyclosporine in the treatment of canine atopic dermatitis. Veterinary Dermatology. 2005;**16**(2):81-86. DOI: 10.1111/j.1365-3164.2005.00435.x

[44] McAtee BB, Cummings KJ, Cook AK, Lidbury JA, Heseltine JC, Willard MD. Opportunistic invasive cutaneous fungal infections associated with administration of cyclosporine to dogs with immune-mediated disease. Journal of Veterinary Internal Medicine. 2017;**31**(6):1724-1729. DOI: 10.1111/jvim.14824

[45] Drucker AM, Ellis AG, Bohdanowicz M, Mashayekhi S, Yiu ZZN, Rochwerg B, et al. Systemic immunomodulatory treatments for patients with atopic dermatitis: A systematic review and network meta-analysis. JAMA Dermatology. 2020;**156**(6):659-667. DOI: 10.1001/jamadermatol.2020.0796

[46] Siegels D, Heratizadeh A, Abraham S, Binnmyr J, Brockow K, Irvine AD, et al. Systemic treatments in the management of atopic dermatitis: A systematic review and meta-analysis. Allergy. 2021;**76**(4):1053-1076. DOI: 10.1111/all.14631

[47] Griffin CE, Hillier A. The ACVD task force on canine atopic dermatitis (XXIV): Allergen-specific immunotherapy. Veterinary Immunology and Immunopathology. 2001;**81**(3-4):363-383. DOI: 10.1016/s0165-2427(01)00348-8

[48] Mueller RS. Update on Allergen Immunotherapy. The Veterinary Clinics of North America. Small Animal Practice. 2019;**49**(1):1-7. DOI: 10.1016/j.cvsm.2018.08.001

[49] Timm K, Mueller RS, Nett-Mettler CS. Long-term effects of intralymphatic immunotherapy (ILIT) on canine atopic dermatitis. Veterinary Dermatology. 2018;**29**(2):123-e49. DOI: 10.1111/vde.12517

[50] Fischer NM, Rostaher A, Favrot C. A comparative study of subcutaneous, intralymphatic and sublingual immunotherapy for the long-term control of dogs with nonseasonal atopic dermatitis. Veterinary Dermatology. 2020;**31**(5):365-e96. DOI: 10.1111/vde.12860

[51] James C, Bernstein DI. Allergen immunotherapy: An updated review of safety. Current Opinion in Allergy Clinical Immunology. 2017;**17**(1):55-59. DOI: 10.1097/ACI.0000000000000335

[52] Tam HH, Calderon MA, Manikam L, Nankervis H, Núñez IG, Williams HC,

et al. Specific allergen immunotherapy for the treatment of atopic eczema: A Cochrane systematic review. Allergy. 2016;**71**(9):1345-1356. DOI: 10.1111/all.12932

[53] Hajdu K, Kapitány A, Dajnoki Z, Soltész L, Baráth S, Hendrik Z, et al. Improvement of clinical and immunological parameters after allergen-specific immunotherapy in atopic dermatitis. Journal of the European Academy of Dermatology and Venereology. 2021;**35**(6):1357-1361. DOI: 10.1111/jdv.17018

[54] DeBoer DJ. The future of immunotherapy for canine atopic dermatitis: A review. Veterinary Dermatology. 2017;**28**(1):25-e6. DOI: 10.1111/vde.12416

[55] Pali-Schöll I, DeBoer DJ, Alessandri C, Seida AA, Mueller RS, Jensen-Jarolim E. Formulations for allergen immunotherapy in human and veterinary patients: New candidates on the horizon. Frontiers in Immunology. 2020;**11**:1697. DOI: 10.3389/fimmu.2020.01697

[56] Tham HL, Olivry T. Determination of the efficacy rate and time-to-efficacy of subcutaneous immunotherapy in dogs with atopic dermatitis. Veterinary Dermatology. 2022;**33**(2):155-e44. DOI: 10.1111/vde.13048

[57] Zubeldia JM, Ferrer M, Dávila I, Justicia JL. Adjuvants in allergen-specific immunotherapy: Modulating and enhancing the immune response. Journal of Investigation Allergology Clinical Immunology. 2019;**29**(2):103-111. DOI: 10.18176/jiaci.0349

[58] Zimmermann J, Goretzki A, Meier C, Wolfheimer S, Lin YJ, Rainer H, et al. Modulation of dendritic cell metabolism by an MPLA-adjuvanted allergen product for specific immunotherapy. Frontiers in Immunology. 2022;**13**:916491. DOI: 10.3389/fimmu.2022.916491

[59] Jonsdottir S, Svansson V, Stefansdottir SB, Schüpbach G, Rhyner C, Marti E, et al. A preventive immunization approach against insect bite hypersensitivity: Intralymphatic injection with recombinant allergens in Alum or Alum and monophosphoryl lipid A. Veterinary Immunology and Immunopathology. 2016;**172**:14-20. DOI: 10.1016/j.vetimm.2016.02.017

[60] Mueller RS, Veir J, Fieseler KV, Dow SW. Use of immunostimulatory liposome-nucleic acid complexes in allergen-specific immunotherapy of dogs with refractory atopic dermatitis - a pilot study. Veterinary Dermatology. 2005;**16**(1):61-68. DOI: 10.1111/j.1365-3164.2005.00426.x

[61] Wagner I, Geh KJ, Hubert M, Winter G, Weber K, Classen J, et al. Preliminary evaluation of cytosine-phosphate-guanine oligodeoxynucleotides bound to gelatine nanoparticles as immunotherapy for canine atopic dermatitis. The Veterinary Record. 2017;**181**(5):118. DOI: 10.1136/vr.104230

[62] Prélaud AR, Fuchs S, Weber K, Winter G, Coester C, Mueller RS. In vitro effects of CpG oligodeoxynucleotides delivered by gelatin nanoparticles on canine peripheral blood mononuclear cells of atopic and healthy dogs - a pilot study. Veterinary Dermatology. 2013;**24**(5):494-e117. DOI: 10.1111/vde.12056

[63] Ricklin Gutzwiller ME, Reist M, Peel JE, Seewald W, Brunet LR, Roosje PJ. 71. Intradermal injection of heat-killed Mycobacterium vaccae in dogs with atopic dermatitis: A multicentre pilot study. Veterinary

Dermatology. 2007;**18**(2):87-93. DOI: 10.1111/j.1365-3164.2007.00579.x

[64] Arkwright PD, David TJ. Effect of Mycobacterium vaccae on atopic dermatitis in children of different ages. The British Journal of Dermatology. 2003;**149**(5):1029-1034. DOI: 10.1111/j.1365-2133.2003.05557.x

[65] Brothers S, Asher MI, Jaksic M, Stewart AW. Effect of a mycobacterium vaccae derivative on pediatric atopic dermatitis: A randomized, controlled trial. Clinical Experiment in Dermatology. 2009;**34**(7):770-775. DOI: 10.1111/j.1365-2230.2008.03153.x

[66] Marro A, Pirles M, et al. Successful 70. immunotherapy of canine flea allergy with injected Actinomycetales preparations. Immunotherapy. 2011;**3**(8):971-978. DOI: 10.2217/imt.11.93

[67] Hendricks AJ, Mills BW, Shi VY. Skin bacterial transplant in atopic dermatitis: Knowns, unknowns and emerging trends. Journal of Dermatological Science. 2019;**95**(2):56-61. DOI: 10.1016/j.jdermsci.2019.07.001

[68] Nakatsuji T, Hata TR, Tong Y, Cheng JY, Shafiq F, Butcher AM, et al. Development of a human skin commensal microbe for bacteriotherapy of atopic dermatitis and use in a phase 1 randomized clinical trial. Nature Medicine. 2021;**27**(4):700-709. DOI: 10.1038/s41591-021-01256-2

[69] Vakharia PP, Silverberg JI. New therapies for atopic dermatitis: Additional treatment classes. Journal of the American Academy of Dermatology. 2018;**78**(3 Suppl. 1):S76-S83. DOI: 10.1016/j.jaad.2017.12.024

[70] Cowan A, Kehner GB, Inan S. Targeting Itch with Ligands Selective for κ Opioid Receptors. Handbook of Experimental Pharmacology. 2015;**226**:291-314. DOI: 10.1007/978-3-662-44,605-8_16

[71] Chiocchetti R, Salamanca G, De Silva M, Gobbo F, Aspidi F, Cunha RZ, et al. Cannabinoid receptors in the inflammatory cells of canine atopic dermatitis. Frontiers in Veterinary Science. 2022;**9**:987132. DOI: 10.3389/fvets.2022.987132

[72] Marsella R, Ahrens K, Sanford R, Trujillo A, Massre D, Soeberdt M, et al. Double blinded, vehicle controlled, crossover study on the efficacy of a topical endocannabinoid membrane transporter inhibitor in atopic Beagles. Archieves in Dermatological Research. 2019;**311**(10):795-800. DOI: 10.1007/s00403-019-01963-4

[73] Loewinger M, Wakshlag JJ, Bowden D, Peters-Kennedy J, Rosenberg A. The effect of a mixed cannabidiol and cannabidiolic acid-based oil on client-owned dogs with atopic dermatitis. Veterinary Dermatology. 2022;**33**(4):329-e77. DOI: 10.1111/vde.13077

[74] Mogi C, Yoshida M, Kawano K, Fukuyama T, Arai T. Effects of cannabidiol without delta-9-tetrahydrocannabinol on canine atopic dermatitis: A retrospective assessment of 8 cases. The Canadian Veterinary Journal. 2022;**63**(4):423-426

[75] Maghfour J, Rietcheck HR, Rundle CW, Runion TM, Jafri ZA, Dercon S, et al. An observational study of the application of a topical cannabinoid gel on sensitive dry skin. Journal of Drugs Dermatology. 2020;**19**(12):1204-1208. DOI: 10.36849/JDD.2020.5464

[76] Palmieri B, Laurino C, Vadalà M. A therapeutic effect of cbd-enriched ointment in inflammatory skin diseases

and cutaneous scars. La Clinica Terapeutica. 2019;**170**(2):e93-e99. DOI: 10.7417/CT.2019.2116

[77] Nickles MA. Lio PA Cannabinoids in Dermatology: Hope or Hype? Cannabis Cannabinoid Research. 2020;**5**(4):279-282. DOI: 10.1089/can.2019.0097

[78] Martins AM, Gomes AL, Vilas Boas I, Marto J, Ribeiro HM. Cannabis-based products for the treatment of skin inflammatory diseases: A Timely Review. Pharmaceuticals (Basel). 2022;**15**(2):210. DOI: 10.3390/ph15020210

[79] Marsella R, Ahrens K, Wilkes R, Soeberdt M, Abels C. Topical κ-opioid receptor agonist asimadoline improves dermatitis in a canine model of atopic dermatitis. Experimental Dermatology. 2022;**31**(4):628-632. DOI: 10.1111/exd.14507

[80] Deeks ED. Difelikefalin: First approval. Drugs. 2022;**81**(16):1937-1944. DOI: 10.1007/s40265-021-01619-6

[81] Chang TT, Stevens SR. Atopic dermatitis: The role of recombinant interferon-gamma therapy. American Journal of Clinical Dermatology. 2002;**3**(3):175-183. DOI: 10.2165/00128071-200,203,030-00004

[82] Mueller RS, Hartmann K. Interferon therapies in small animals. Veterinary Journal. 2021;**271**:105648. DOI: 10.1016/j.tvjl.2021.105648

[83] Iwasaki T, Hasegawa A. A randomized comparative clinical trial of recombinant canine interferon-gamma (KT-100) in atopic dogs using antihistamine as control. Veterinary Dermatology. 2006;**17**(3):195-200. DOI: 10.1111/j.1365-3164.2006.00519.x

[84] Yasukawa K, Saito S, Kubo T, Shibasaki Y, Yamaoka K, Hachimura H, et al. Low-dose recombinant canine interferon-gamma for treatment of canine atopic dermatitis: An open randomized comparative trial of two doses. Veterinary Dermatology. 2010;**21**(1):42-49. DOI: 10.1111/j.1365-3164.2009.00764.x

[85] Carlotti DN, Boulet M, Ducret J, Machicote G, Jasmin P, Rème CA, et al. The use of recombinant omega interferon therapy in canine atopic dermatitis: A double-blind controlled study. Veterinary Dermatology. 2009;**20**(5-6):405-411. DOI: 10.1111/j.1365-3164.2009.00848.x

[86] Litzlbauer P, Weber K, Mueller RS. Oral and subcutaneous therapy of canine atopic dermatitis with recombinant feline interferon omega. Cytokine. 2014;**66**(1):54-59. DOI: 10.1016/j.cyto.2013.12.001

[87] Breno C et al. Recombinant human interferon-α14 for the treatment of canine allergic pruritic disease in eight dogs. Veterinary Record Open. 2021;**8**(1):e6. DOI: 10.1002/vro2.6

[88] Daltro SRT, Meira CS, Santos IP, Ribeiro Dos Santos R, MBP S. Mesenchymal stem cells and atopic dermatitis: A review. Cytokine Frontiers in Cell Developmental Biology. 2020;**14**(8):326. DOI: 10.3389/fcell.2020.00326

[89] Najera J, Hao J. Recent advance in mesenchymal stem cells therapy for atopic dermatitis. Journal of Cellular Biochemistry. 2022. DOI: 10.1002/jcb.30365

[90] Klinger C. Mesenchymal stem cells: A potential therapy for canine atopic dermatitis? The Veterinary Record. 2018;**183**(21):651-653. DOI: 10.1136/vr.k4985

[91] Hezam K, Mo R, Wang C, Liu Y, Li Z. Anti-inflammatory Effects

of Mesenchymal Stem Cells and their Secretomes in Pneumonia. Current Pharmaceutical Biotechnology. 2022;**23**(9):1153-1167. DOI: 10.2174/1389201022666210907115126

[92] Al-Ghadban S, Bunnell BA. Adipose tissue-derived stem cells. Immunomodulatory Effects and Therapeutic Potential Physiology (Bethesda). 2020;**35**(2):125-133. DOI: 10.1152/physiol.00021.2019

[93] Hall MN, Rosenkrantz WS, Hong JH, Griffin CE, Mendelsohn CM. Evaluation of the potential use of adipose-derived mesenchymal stromal cells in the treatment of canine atopic dermatitis: A pilot study. Veterinary Therapy. 2010;**11**(2):E1-E14

[94] Villatoro AJ, Hermida-Prieto M, Fernández V, Fariñas F, Alcoholado C, Rodríguez-García MI, et al. Allogeneic adipose-derived mesenchymal stem cell therapy in dogs with refractory atopic dermatitis: Clinical efficacy and safety. The Veterinary Record. 2018;**183**(21):654. DOI: 10.1136/vr.104867

[95] de Oliveira RF, Malard PF, Brunel HDSS, Paludo GR, de Castro MB, da Silva PHS, et al. Canine atopic dermatitis attenuated by mesenchymal stem cells. Journal of Advanced Veterinary Animal Research. 2020;**7**(3):554-565. DOI: 10.5455/javar.2020.g453

[96] Kaur G, Ramirez A, Xie C, Clark D, Dong C, Maki C, et al. A double-blinded placebo-controlled evaluation of adipose-derived mesenchymal stem cells in treatment of canine atopic dermatitis. Veterinary Research Communications. 2022;**46**(1):251-260. DOI: 10.1007/s11259-021-09853-9

[97] Enciso N, Amiel J, Pando J, Enciso J. Multidose intramuscular allogeneic adipose stem cells decrease the severity of canine atopic dermatitis: A pilot study. Veterinary Record. 2019;**12**(11):1747-1754. DOI: 10.14202/vetworld.2019.1747-1754

[98] Lo Sicco C, Reverberi D, Balbi C, Ulivi V, Principi E, Pascucci L, et al. Mesenchymal stem cell-derived extracellular vesicles as mediators of anti-inflammatory effects: Endorsement of macrophage polarization stem cells. Translational Medicine. 2017;**6**(3):1018-1028. DOI: 10.1002/sctm.16-0363

[99] Cho BS, Kim JO, Ha DH, Yi YW. Exosomes derived from human adipose tissue-derived mesenchymal stem cells alleviate atopic dermatitis. Stem Cell Research Therapy. 2018;**9**(1):187. DOI: 10.1186/s13287-018-0939-5